Six Months to Live

Six Months to Live

LEARNING FROM A YOUNG MAN
WITH CANCER

DANIEL HALLOCK

 THE PLOUGH PUBLISHING HOUSE

06 05 04 03 02 01 00   11 10 9 8 7 6 5 4 3 2 1

Front Cover Photograph: © Andrzej Lech/Graphistock

A catalog record for this book
is available from the British Library.

Library of Congress Cataloging-in-Publication Data

Hallock, D. (Daniel)
  Six months to live : learning from a young man with cancer / Daniel
William Hallock.
    p. cm.
  ISBN 0-87486-903-x
  1. Gauger, Matt, d. 2000–Health. 2.
Lymphoma–Patients–Pennsylvania–Biography. I. Title.
  RC280.L9 H347 2001
  362.1'9699446'0092–dc21

                                          00-012514

Printed in the USA

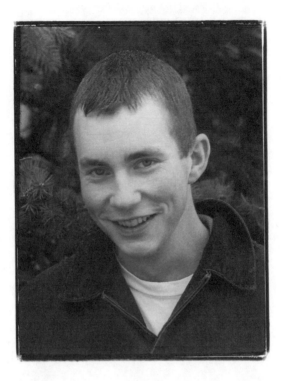

"He was no sage or angel but a person who, under the stress of terrible agony, learned to accept being weak without being ashamed."

HERMANN HESSE
"PETER CAMENZIND"

CONTENTS

PREFACE IX

1. THE BLOW 1

2. GOBBLER 15

3. CYNTHIA 26

4. LIFE WITH CHEMO 39

5. BACK TO THE FRONT 54

6. LEARNING TO LET GO 69

7. BEFORE MORNING 82

8. TIES THAT BIND 100

9. NEW SEEDS 120

CODA 133

PREFACE

AS WE ROSE from our chairs at the end of the
service, which was held outdoors, six men – including
Matt's dad, Randy, and his brother, Nick – picked up
his wooden casket. Several friends had made it by
hand and painted it white, and it was covered with
hundreds of lovingly scrawled messages.

After the pallbearers came a long, silent train:
eight hundred friends, family members, relatives,
classmates, and fellow church members, winding past
Matt's old school, past the basketball court where he'd
played, and the playing field, and up the valley.

We came out of the woods and into the burial
ground, and the crowd filled the sunlit lawn. Matt's
casket was lowered. A dozen peers stepped forward,
shovels in hand. Tears blinded a few as they threw

earth into the grave, and now and then someone missed completely.

A guitar strummed, and Springsteen's gentle rasp vibrated from a speaker behind the crowd. Cynthia, Matt's wife of five months, had found her husband crying as he listened to the same recording a week or so before. She had cried, too, when she heard the lyrics, and decided it should be played at his funeral:

> Tonight my bag is packed;
> tomorrow I'll walk these tracks
> that will lead me across the border.
>
> Tomorrow my love and I
> will sleep 'neath auburn skies
> somewhere across the border.
>
> For you I'll build a house
> high up on a grassy hill
> Somewhere across the border.
>
> Where pain and memory –
> pain and memory – have been stilled
> there across the border
>
> and sweet blossoms fill the air,
> pastures of gold and green
> roll down into cool clear waters,
>
> and in your arms 'neath the open skies
> I'll kiss the sorrow from your eyes
> there across the border.

For what are we
without hope in our hearts
that someday we'll drink from God's blessed waters

and eat the fruit from the vine?
I know love and fortune will be mine
somewhere across the border.

Now Cynthia – a widow at twenty-one – placed a bouquet of long-stemmed roses at the head of the grave, a look of triumph playing across her face. As she straightened, two little girls ran forward to add their flowers. Suddenly the crowd surged forward from all sides, and in minutes the grave was a mound of bright bouquets.

Roses had been brought for onlookers who didn't have their own flowers, and two still stood in a pitcher on the ground. Dave, a close friend who had mentored Matt during his high school years, took one and placed it on the heap. Howard, another friend, took the remaining one and did the same, before breaking into sobs. Cynthia tried to comfort him.

Across the circle, someone began "We Shall Overcome." Eight hundred voices joined in, catching with emotion. As a young woman put it later, "I will never forget how that song rang out. It was a language we could all understand. It was the holiest moment I have ever experienced." "Everyone was breaking down," another remembered. "But it wasn't because we were sad. We weren't crying over Matt's death. We were crying for joy and awe."

Standing there in the enormous, largely youthful crowd, I had noted the same thing: unlike so many other funerals, this one was neither unbearably heavy nor depressing, but strangely joyful. Part of it was the setting: Matt comes from the Bruderhof, the religious order I joined eleven years ago. In our community death – like everything else, from work, worship, and meals, to care of children and the elderly – is shared, and we live on communally owned grounds that might best be described as a monastery for families.

Like Matt and his family, who came to the Bruderhof two years before me, I grew up in a typical middle-class home, where the subject of death – like illness, grief, heartache, or other sources of anxiety – was assiduously avoided. It's not that a conscious taboo existed. But "negative" life experiences were rarely, if ever, discussed outside the family. We simply didn't "go there," conversation-wise.

As a working adult, I found the same silence, the same walls carefully constructed around each personal life. When the wife of an engineer at my firm – a kindly man I regarded as a mentor – came down with cancer, he brushed off every expression of sympathy. It seemed as though he was obeying some unspoken code whereby vulnerability is seen as instability, and

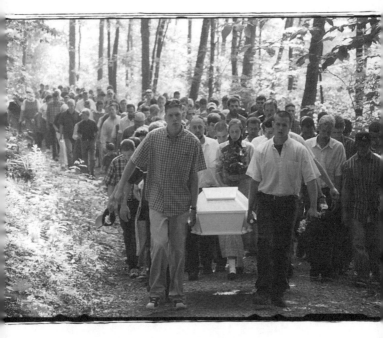

On the way to the burial

pain as weakness. Obviously he couldn't afford to be associated with either. He had to remain strong.

I know Ed loved his wife dearly, but to this day I am amazed at the lengths he went to detach himself from her suffering, at least on the job. One day he told me rather matter-of-factly that his wife's tumor had burst; a few days later he walked into the office and announced that his wife had died that morning. I was incredulous that he had come to work – though it's possible there was no one at home for him to talk to. On the other hand, the way he dealt with losing his spouse was hardly out of sync with the way everything else was dealt with in our workaday world. There was never any lack of camaraderie, but it was only a façade. When the chips were down, you kept a lid on things – no matter how much you were hurting.

The anguish of Matt's loss, on the other hand, was carried not only by his widow, his parents, and hers, but by an entire community that surrounded and upheld them. Moreover, it was accepted and embraced and plumbed for meaning in a way I can't imagine happening anywhere else. As Matt's grandmother, Janet, wrote afterward, the funeral and the days preceding it meant more to her "than all the church services I have ever attended. What should have been a horrendous experience was turned into a celebration of life, and of thanks to God for what he did in Matt's life."

Perhaps that was the biggest difference between this funeral, which one of Matt's friends unhesitatingly pronounced "incredible, wonderful" and the ones I had avoided in my younger days. There were at least three. Two high school friends were killed in highway crashes – one of them a guy I'd been hanging out with just a few nights before. We'd talked late into the night about our plans for the future, and the next thing I knew, he was dead. He had driven home drunk from a nightclub at two in the morning and ended up wrapped around a tree. Another friend died of stomach cancer. He spent the last months of his life in his house, ashamed of his illness, and too insecure to go out. In short, I have (like everyone else I know) my own litany of the dead: friends or family members who died suddenly, or without hope or comfort – each one an unwelcome reminder of mortality and a threat to dreams of a long, prosperous life, or at least a happy and "fulfilled" one.

As a teen (and later, as a twenty-something) I had my ways of trying to shrug such reminders off, of keeping them at an arm's length and moving on. Mostly I made light of it. "Live fast, die young, and leave a beautiful corpse" was my motto – though of course I reserved it for those unfortunate blips in time when death "happened" to someone else.

It almost happened to me. I was walking home with a group of fellow undergrads from a rock concert on campus. We'd taken a familiar short-cut. But we were stoned and only vaguely aware of just how close it ran along the edge of a deep gorge.

Friends tell me that I was there one second and gone the next. I myself remember nothing at all, except that when I woke up I was lying on my back looking up at a sky full of stars. I cried out, twice, and the second time I was answered by a friend some twenty feet above me. Reassured that I was still alive, he raced off to get help and came back with an acquaintance who was a climber. Together they lowered a rope and hauled me back up to the path.

My friends were ecstatic. Someone lit a joint, and we took stock of what had happened. I'd stumbled off the cliff and fallen onto a ledge about three feet wide – the only one of its kind along a mile-long stretch of the gorge. Had I fallen anywhere else, I would never have survived. As it was, I had landed flat on my back, on moss, and I didn't have a single scratch or bruise.

Back at the dorms, we partied up a storm. Yet as we laughed I caught a classmate staring at me as if I were some ghost returned from the dead. I suppose I felt like one. I had cheated death, but only by inches.

Looking back I see now that by mocking the incident, instead of letting it shatter me, I avoided its impact and missed a rare opportunity to examine my life – its meaning, its direction, its purpose, its demands.

But this book is not about me. It's about Matt, whom death snatched at twenty-two – though he also cheated it, as you'll see – and about the lessons his last six months on earth could have for you, if you are open to them.

On the surface, Matt's story is just one of countless inexplicably "unfair" tragedies. Yet for those of us who were close to him – as for anyone who is close to any death, no matter how "normal" – it needs to be told, because of the rare way in which it has already been lived and shared by so many. To quote a handful of the messages on his casket:

> Matt – your death showed me that God is real. Thanx for being there, Cathy.

> Nothing profound, man. I'll see you when I get there – Eric.

> Matt, I'll never forget throwing a football with you before you got sick. Your life has challenged me to live each day as if it's my last. See you, Allen.

> Matt, thank you for being real and not trying to be someone else. You taught me a lot. Suzy.

> Matt – Your life disturbed me, in a good way. I'll always hold a place for you in my life. Make sure to visit. Love you man, Luke.

> You've put a longing in my heart, and I pray it will stay there – Jenna.

No matter how, where, and when we live, each of us will one day have to pass through the doorway of death – and through suffering as well. Through Matt's illness and death, those of us who knew him felt as if we were allowed a glimpse through that door and given insights from "across the border" – insights that may yet determine the course of our lives, even if we cannot articulate them. It is as if that door, long shut, has suddenly been opened, and we are no longer afraid to enter the rooms beyond it. Perhaps this book can open the same door for you.

D. H.
December 2000

1

THE BLOW

SUMMER 1999 was a whirlwind for Randy and Linda Gauger. In June they flew to Littleton, Colorado, to house-sit for a couple whose daughter had been killed in the recent Columbine massacre; in July they returned home to the Bruderhof in Farmington, Pennsylvania, where their oldest son, Matt, lived. In August they were in the air once again, this time heading for Danthonia, the community's new branch in Australia.

Expecting to be away for a minimum of several months – Randy was to oversee the legal affairs of the new venture – they asked Jonathan, a fellow Bruderhof member and family physician, if he would mind looking out for Matt while they were away. (Nick, their second child, had left Farmington after high school and was starting his third year of college in Pittsburgh.)

After his parents left, Matt began eating breakfasts with Jonathan and his wife, and he was soon stopping by to read bedtime stories to their children as well. During the day he worked in the IS (information services) department at Community Playthings, the Bruderhof's main business. Life was unremarkable – until a memorable Saturday in late November. As Jonathan later recounted:

> We were finishing up the breakfast dishes on the 20th when Matt told me that he had noticed lumps in his groin two days earlier. He wondered whether they could ever indicate a serious problem. I said no, because they are almost always associated with infections, and infections can be taken care of with antibiotics. But I told him that if he was having pain, he should keep me in touch. The same evening the phone rang at six o'clock; it was Matt, and he asked me to bring a hefty dose of Motrin for him when I came to the community dining room that night. He met me at the door and snatched the Motrin from my hands. He was very uncomfortable. At ten o'clock he came by our apartment and begged to be examined, so I took him to my office and did so. He said he had a great deal of pain in his left groin and was sure it was a hernia. On examination I found several tender, marble-sized lymph nodes in the left groin. I recommended a high dose of Motrin, but

did not start an antibiotic as there was no sign of infection on the left leg or foot.

On Sunday Matt felt fairly well. On Monday, however, while driving home alone from Pittsburgh, where he had dropped off a friend at the airport, he was in such pain that he debated calling home and asking for someone to come pick him up. At home, he went straight to the doctor's office. A second exam showed nothing new, but Jonathan started him on an antibiotic anyway. That night at the members' meeting – a daily gathering for dialogue and worship – Jonathan noticed that Matt sat in the back row, slouching to keep his groin comfortable.

Tuesday afternoon Matt's pain worsened, and he complained of backache. At nine in the evening, Jonathan found him lying on the living room couch. Matt begged to be re-examined. Once again they went to the office, and once again no significant problem was found. Jonathan offered Ultram, a stronger painkiller, but Matt still called him after midnight, asking if it was okay to up the frequency of his dosage.

On Wednesday Matt was seen by a specialist at the local hospital. Nothing new was found, but the doctor felt he should continue the antibiotic. Matt was reassured and spoke of canceling the follow-up appointment.

At story time that night, Jonathan's four-year-old Alan was hurt when Matt wouldn't let him sit on his lap. At bedtime, however, he prayed that Matt would soon feel better. It was then that it first crossed Jonathan's mind that Matt's problem might be something serious.

On Thursday night Matt was so uncomfortable that Jonathan had to give him sleeping pills at one a.m.; by breakfast the next day, he was complaining of severe back pain. By Friday evening he was in such agony that Jonathan stopped the Ultram and put him on codeine, but when he asked Matt if he'd called his parents about the last four days, Matt shot back, "Why should I tell them anything? They'll only worry about me." Jonathan worried, though. Twelve years earlier, while treating a cancer patient in New York, he'd written in his journal: "She began her week on Tylenol, and ended it on morphine." Matt, too, had started the week the same way, and he was ending it on narcotics.

Back in Matt's room, a handful of friends was trying to cheer Matt up with a little good-natured ribbing. "Matt," Tim intoned, "I've been asked to break the news to you. You have…cancer." Everyone laughed, but Matt winged a book and pair of socks at Tim and told everyone to get the hell out of his room.

By mid-morning the next day, Matt was in the local hospital for a CT scan of his abdomen and

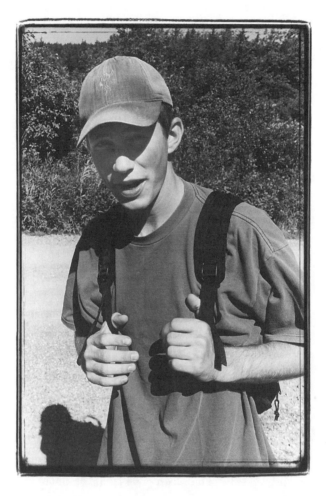

Hiking in West Virginia

pelvis. To Jonathan's shock, the scan revealed enlarged lymph nodes deep in the abdomen. Infection was still a possibility, the radiologist assured him, but there were two other possibilities as well: metastatic testicular carcinoma or a lymphoma. Jonathan broke the news to Matt, and on the way home they discussed a plan of action: continue the painkillers and antibiotics, but if there's no improvement in a day or two, biopsy a node from the left groin. The hours that followed are burned into Jonathan's memory:

> Matt moped around our house, lying on the couch or on my son's bed, crouching in funny positions, pacing the floor, trying to get comfortable. I offered to do something more – to take him back to the hospital, to do *something* – but he was adamant that we had to "give it some time" before proceeding further.
>
> Matt joined our family for dinner. Around eleven I went to his room to check on him and found that he had a fever. This worried me, because nocturnal fevers are sometimes associated with malignancy, so I decided then and there that Matt needed to be under closer observation. I brought him to our apartment and settled him in an extra room.
>
> Around midnight he called through our bedroom door to say that he wanted to take his narcotic again. I reminded him that the usual prescription

was "every four hours," and that he had just had a tablet one hour go, but I let him take another. An hour later he was banging on the door again. This time I gave him a shot of Demerol. It did nothing to relieve his condition. By three a.m. – after another dose of Demerol – he was inconsolable, alternately pacing the living room and curling up on the floor, weeping. I called the hospital, and we were soon in the car, heading down the highway to the emergency room...

Halfway around the globe, Randy and Linda were sitting at the phone, trying to get through to the Bruderhof in Pennsylvania. Someone had relayed a message that Matt was sick, but Linda was sure it was a mistake. "Matt never got sick," she recalled. "Nick was the one always coming down with something strange. I almost wanted it to be Nick, because I had been with him when he had pain, or when he was nervous and scared. I know how he reacts and handles things. But how would Matt deal with it? He had no experience with pain." Little did she know what he was going through that very moment – one wave of pain after another, so brutal and searing that before long his morphine injections were abandoned in favor of a continuous intravenous drip.

On Sunday Tim visited Matt with Brian, another friend, and they decided to stay at the hospital overnight. The experience was pure hell, but Tim felt he was doing penance for his joke two days before:

> I'll tell you, it was the most agonizing hours I've ever spent with anyone. Matt was getting morphine shots when I arrived, but he was in such pain that they didn't help. Every half hour he'd start writhing around in bed. He was fidgeting with his sheets, biting his lips, and drawing deep breaths. Then he'd get up, because he couldn't sit any more, and pace wildly or crawl around on the floor. He was bellowing, "Oh God, *please* help me!"
>
> Sometimes his pain was so bad that he would bend over double and claw at the walls. I've never seen anyone in such agony. He'd try one position after the next – squatting on the floor, sitting on the heater, lying on the bed. Every position caused excruciating pain.
>
> At one point Matt was lying in bed, and he looked at me and said, "You know, Tim, it would *really* suck if this was cancer, wouldn't it?" I said, "Yeah, it would." Later a football game came on. Matt said, "Just so you guys know, I am not the entertainment. Watch the TV."

But they couldn't. Brian remembers:

> For six long hours we sat next to Matt in relative silence. There's nothing worse than sitting there helplessly, watching someone's face contort with

pain and knowing you can't do a thing to alleviate it. We put our arms around him and rubbed his back and told him to hang in there. We wiped his face and forehead and adjusted his pillow. We gave him water to drink and tried to tidy up the room. When a nurse brought him prune juice (he had trouble going to the bathroom) he tried to laugh, but the next moment he was balling up his sheet and biting at it in pain.

During one of his worst episodes – he was lying on the floor, gasping for breath – his parents called in from Australia, and he was saying, "No, I'm all right; I'm fine." That's when I started crying.

On Monday, Matt's second day in the hospital, he underwent a bone marrow aspiration. During the procedure, a hollow, eighth-inch bit is drilled into the patient's hip bone – first on one side of the base of the spine, and then on the other. Following this, suction is applied in order to extract marrow for testing. Jonathan calls that moment the mule kick – the point at which the patient, who is normally howling in pain despite local anesthesia, will suddenly "go through the ceiling." Jonathan remembered later:

> Matt was very dubious about the whole thing, if only because it would require lying flat on his belly for a long time, a position he had not been able to attain in more than a week. As it was, the 45-minute procedure was sheer hell. Matt was kicking

and screaming. I told him to squeeze my fingers, and squeeze them he did! My fingers ached for days afterward, and my knuckles were purple and bruised. Matt's pillowcase was so saturated with tears that I could have literally wrung it out. And I cannot say how many tears *I* shed, to see him in this condition. If anyone thinks he can tolerate pain, he should try a bone marrow aspiration.

Jonathan drove in to see Matt multiple times over the next few days:

One time I dropped by and found Frank and another guy pacing the room with Matt. He would yell, and they would yell with him; he would cry and they would cry. He would grasp their hands, embrace them in bear hugs and squeeze them till they could hardly breathe. Then he'd collapse on the bed and fall asleep.

Another time when I came in, Frank was sitting on the floor. His face was beet red from hours of crying and rubbing his eyes. Matt was dozing peacefully, but Frank said that every time his fever spiked, his pain would drive him up the wall, and he'd be completely out of control for the next hour or so. Frank had been through two of these episodes when I found him, and he was an emotional wreck.

In one sense, the young men who endured Matt's first days of agony with him were only observers; in another, they were – as one of them put it later – being "laid low" along with him. Suddenly, life had been stripped to the bare essentials, to a battle for survival. "It totally threw me," recalls Frank. "Matt had been living a normal life just *days* before all this! Now he was hooked up to monitors and IV lines and needed help getting in and out of a bathroom."

Jonathan noted the same thing, but what really struck him was the change in Matt's demeanor. Just one week ago he had been a capable, happy-go-lucky adult. Now he was more like a frightened, clinging child:

> It was striking how quickly his confidence was toppled by his pain. He willingly let me – no, begged me – pull him up in bed, smooth out his sheets, change his pajamas, bathe him, rub his legs, scratch his back, hold a glass of water to his mouth, run a damp washcloth between his toes, and dry his feet with a towel.
>
> When I accompanied him to the OR for a lymph node excision, he was quite frightened, as he had never undergone an operation before. He asked a hundred questions over the next hour and begged me not to leave his side. I promised him I wouldn't. I also reminded him of a conversation we had had the night before: that no matter how things turned out, we had to pray that it would be according to God's will.

On Monday Matt asked me point blank whether I thought he had cancer. I told him that it was indeed looking more and more like it. He sat silent, aghast, and then looked me straight in the eye, tears streaming down his cheeks: "Do you think I will die before New Year's?" "Only God knows," I told him.

It was at this point that I decided to tell Matt that the community had bought tickets for his parents, and that they were probably on their way from Sydney as we spoke. "That's bad!" he grimaced. "It is," I agreed. "But you *are* in a bad way, and we have to face it and fight it." He then said resignedly that if his parents were coming home all the way from Australia, it must be clear that he had cancer. All I could do was remind him that there was no firm diagnosis, and that there was nothing I knew that he didn't.

The next days were a blur. Tuesday morning the pathology reports had come in: Matt had lymphoma, and it appeared to be an anaplastic, large-cell type. Further, the cancer seemed to have spread from the abdomen to the chest. At noon Matt was transferred by ambulance to the university hospital in nearby Morgantown, West Virginia. Later that afternoon an oncologist came by. His report confirmed everyone's worst fears: Matt had anaplastic, large-cell lymphoma. Chemo could help him, but it would have to be started the very next day.

Meanwhile, Randy and Linda were on the way home, flying first from rural New South Wales to Sydney, then on to Los Angeles – a flight of twenty-one hours – then to New York, and finally to Morgantown. As Randy remembers the grueling trip:

> We had a five-hour layover in Sydney and were already totally exhausted. We hadn't slept for two nights. At first the airline couldn't find our tickets, but after a few calls back and forth, they located them. An agent noticed how distraught we were and asked why we were going home. When she found out, she arranged for us to travel business class.
>
> We knew that Matt was having tests but had not heard the outcome, so I called home. I broke down on the phone when I heard the diagnosis, and when I returned to Linda, I was barely able to talk. I said something like, "It's cancer and it's bad." We both just sat there and cried. We were unable to talk for a long time. Later we got up and walked aimlessly around the airport, tears falling from our faces. Linda finally asked me if we would get home in time to see Matt. I told her I didn't know. "Numb" is the only way I can describe my feelings at the time.
>
> Once in the air, we talked very little. We mostly held hands, and cried. I do remember talking about how good it was that Matt was in the arms of our church, with people who knew him – with brothers and sisters. That was a tremendous comfort. We also

read off and on from a little book we'd brought
along, *Now Is Eternity.* We needed to hold on to
something other than our fear.

Back at the hospital, Matt's fever was spiking again.
More blood was drawn, and additional morphine was
administered, along with intravenous steroids. Matt
mumbled, "Sure hope Dad and Mom don't see me
like this." But a few minutes later they did. In Linda's
words :

> Matt was in bed when we walked in, an IV pump
> in his arm. We hugged and cried and told him how
> glad we were to be there with him, and he said he
> was glad we'd come. There was little else to say.
> Later we went down the street to a motel room the
> community had booked for us to try to get some
> rest. We couldn't. Everywhere we looked, there were
> flowers, food, and greetings from brothers and sis-
> ters at home. We stayed up for two hours reading
> them, and the love they expressed overwhelmed us.
> But Matt's situation kept tugging at us too. Why
> was this happening? We still couldn't really believe
> it or take it in. Our son – *our son* – had cancer.

2

GOBBLER

"NOT MATT." That was the most common reaction as the news spread. True, it might have been predictable – the word "cancer" has a way of stopping people in their tracks – but somehow, at least to those who knew him, Matt seemed an especially unlikely victim. When people thought of Matt, they thought easy-come, easy-go; they thought of his moves on the court, his loopy grin, his ability to catch every word of a song the first or second time he heard it on the radio. Hannah, a high school classmate, thought of his big mouth:

> A lot of people called him Gauger, but to some of us he was always Gobbler. We called him that because he never stopped talking. He'd salivate as he talked,

and wipe away the spit with his hand, and laugh, and go on blabbering. Whenever you were in a crowd, you'd always hear Matt above everybody else, talking his head off. And he was so animated. He had this crazy laugh that sent him lurching over double and slapping his knees.

Ben, another classmate, has similar memories:

I'll never forget the time he and Zach tried to "kill" Chet and me with a blunted putty knife in the school woodshop. Or the time he locked me in the car wash and soaked me over and over. One time he even tried to wrestle our teacher. Matt fought like crazy, talked like crazy, laughed like crazy, and was a pain. He was a big, geeky kid.

He had these annoying one-liners, like: "Insert foot in mouth, then chew." Or he'd clutch his throat with one hand and try to pull it off with the other. He had a way of walking that pushed you off the edge of the road, and won the reputation of being a tailgater – a guy who follows you around because he wants to be your friend. I remember trying desperately to shake him. Yet I'm sure it never crossed his mind to think bad of me, and in other ways he was the winningest.

Matt had a killer one-handed, no-arc jumper which ruled the basketball court. We called it the snakey, because his wrist kind of snapped when the ball left his hands. That fade-away jump shot from the right corner was all net all the time, and almost impossible to block. In softball, his long hard drives down the third-base line were completely predictable, but damaging.

Matt made friends in high school long before most of us knew where the bathrooms were. Guys liked him because friendship was more important to him than grades. He'd spend all his time in homeroom goofing around and still pull tests in the upper 90's. If not? Well, there were things more important in life.

And the girls…all of them liked him. I remember thinking 'Gosh, what a flirt!' But it wasn't like he ever tried to come on to someone. He was just a people person. He couldn't have cared less who he was talking to.

Matt had tremendous drive. One time in high school he was mowing this huge hay field, and a stray dog ate his lunch while he was on the tractor. He spent fourteen hours in the sun that day without food or water, and came home in the evening looking real pale. But he got the job done. I think he got that sense of responsibility from his parents.

Matt loved his parents, by the way. He never showed any signs of embarrassment over them, even when we teased him about his barn chores and the other things his dad made him do – like getting up early to muck out the stalls. He'd come on the bus smelling like manure. If you didn't like it, tough cookies.

Matt wouldn't take abuse from anyone, but he would also be the first to stand up when someone else was disrespected. I'll never forget how he stood up for Maya – she was the only black student on our bus – on the way home from school one day. Someone was harassing her or something, and he got up in the aisle with his fists clenched. The driver had to pull over and stop the bus.

Eileen, a college classmate, remembers Matt's generosity – especially the time he gave her his books from the previous semester and told her to sell them at the university book exchange. "Go buy yourself something with the money," he said.

Matt's brother, Nick, of course, has earlier memories:

Matt and I fought a lot, though I guess siblings are always like that, and it wasn't like something separated us. But he was a good teaser; he knew what would make me upset.

When we were little we used to play with this kid named Brody, another guy, Matt's age, called Reid, and a girl my age, named Amy. I would tease Brody, and then everyone else would tease me. Reid

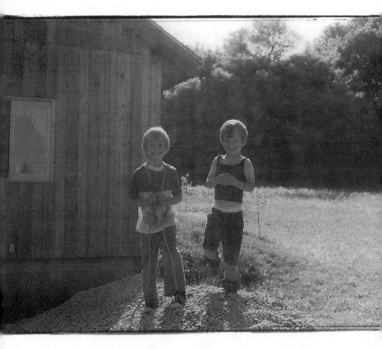

On the farm in Minnesota

and Matt would trip me or something and I'd fall. Then I'd throw huge temper tantrums. It wasn't funny. I'd get so angry, I'd pick up a rock or a tree branch – something from the woods – and I'd just heave it at Matt!

Other times when I got fed up with their teasing I'd run over to our tree house, where I'd stockpiled some stones, and I'd climb up and throw them at Matt as hard as I could.

But those are good memories. Even though Matt would always send me off crying because I was hurt or because he'd teased me too much, when things got really serious he was always there for me. This continued even in high school. I think I must have made a good target for people to go after or pick on, but Matt would stand up to anyone for me.

Later, Matt's main claim to fame was his knack for getting out of a scrape – the water fight that turned into a brawl, or the time he broke a rearview mirror in a moving car. No matter how sticky the situation, he seemed able to lawyer his way out of it or disarm his challenger with a guffaw. As Megan, another classmate, puts it, "Even if he was in a tight spot, he acted as if he was in control – which often helped him get out of it. Besides, he was always so likable…"

Despite this reputation, however (or perhaps because of it), no one who knew Matt will forget the time he was really in a pinch and didn't try to wiggle out of it. It happened in late 1996, at a warehouse leased by the Bruderhof. Officially, Matt and a buddy were doing their job – nighttime security. In reality, they spent the night drinking and wound up thoroughly hung over. By morning the empties were gone, the floor mopped. But the room still reeked of vomit, and there were other telltale signs.

Confronted, Matt owned up, not only to getting drunk but also to stealing the alcohol in question. Further, he apologized at a community members' meeting the next day, volunteering that "my life has been going down the drain, and I can't fix it by myself." "I need God in my life," Matt admitted to the gathering, "and I need your help. I ask for your forgiveness, and I thank everyone who has taken the time to speak with me and find out how I'm doing."

Though the matter was quickly laid to rest, it seemed to be a turning point for Matt; from then on, some acquaintances say, he began to take life more seriously and to engage in fewer antics. Others disagree. According to them, the real change came later, after Matt left the Bruderhof for a five-month stint at the Open Door, an Atlanta outreach that runs a soup kitchen and a shelter for the homeless.

In a November 1997 letter to his parents, he wrote:

This morning I served breakfast and noticed several people who must have AIDS. They're obviously in pretty bad shape but are still out on the street…A lot of people are sick with colds, too, and tired from having to walk around all the time. Every night we give out blankets to whoever needs them. The homeless aren't allowed to sit in public places; the police run them off if they have no permanent address. But it's pretty amazing that almost every one of them is cheerful, or at least makes the effort to look cheerful, when coming through the food line. You know that they probably didn't get much sleep last night, and that it was down to about 35 degrees. They have every reason to be upset. They don't really have anything to live for. Yet still they smile at you and say good morning. It sure challenges me.

Last Sunday we had a pretty good meeting. The theme of the sermon was John the Baptist and his call to repentance. It sounded really familiar, but sort of refreshing…

A few months later, Matt returned to the Bruderhof and asked to become a member. He was baptized – a step that signifies full membership in the community – in June 1998. A few days before this, in a meeting where he and several other peers were asked to explain why they wanted to be baptized, he said:

I need to find a relationship with God and with everybody here…I've been a rotten example. I am determined not to talk a lot, but to show my faith in deeds. Up till now…I've been pretending to be focused on God when I really wasn't; I made people think I was a Christian, or that I was dedicated to this way of life. I haven't been. That's where I'm going to change…

It was this same honesty about himself that touched many people a year and a half later, in the days that followed Matt's return home from the hospital. Understandably, most patients who have just been diagnosed with a serious illness are primarily concerned with their physical condition. Matt, too, was worried about that, and peppered his doctors with questions – What was the cause of the lymphoma? How effective was the treatment supposed to be? What were his chances of survival? What did this or that medical term mean? But his overriding concern was his spiritual state. It was, Jonathan recalls, as if Matt sensed that his life had taken an irreversible turn, and that no matter what the outcome, he needed to set his life in order.

I dropped by Matt's room two days after he'd been discharged and noticed that he'd been crying. I asked him what was up and he told me, in brief, that he had had a long talk with his dad, and that he felt he had to deepen his life. He said there were things on his conscience that he needed to tell someone about. He also said he felt "scared and lonely." I suggested that he try to get out of the house in the next few days, even if he felt rotten. Maybe that would help. But he just looked past me and said, "My relationship with God is not what it should be." I assured him that all of us needed to deepen our lives, not just him, and that his illness was helping us all to realize our need for God. Matt just lay there with big wet eyes, staring straight ahead, absorbing the gravity of his personal situation. Looking at him I suddenly realized that each of us needs such a moment.

Two weeks later, Matt e-mailed Christoph, a trusted friend, and the Elder of the Bruderhof:

There is a passage in the Bible [James 5:13–16] which is very important to me right now. It talks about telling each other your sins so that your prayers will be heard and answered. Making sure that all of my sins are confessed and forgiven, and asking forgiveness of people whom I've hurt, has never been so important to me as it is right now… more important than physical healing. When your need for God outweighs your need to appear flawless in front of the people around you, repentance becomes something you long for, not dread. I experienced this very personally when I came home from the hospital. I knew it was literally a matter of life or death to straighten out my relationship with God if I was going to get through my illness.

In the weeks and months that followed, Matt sent numerous such e-mails to Christoph, and the answers he received in return were a source of deep comfort to him. So were their conversations and phone calls. To recount just one, in Christoph's words:

I told him that having cancer means having one's personal power dismantled, and that perhaps God was trying to speak to him through it. I also reminded him that he had everything going for him up till now: he was young and strong and handsome and gifted. He had the world by the tail. But now God was saying, "Uh-uh. You're no good to me." God had allowed him to have cancer. It was a terrific blow – there was no question. But perhaps God couldn't use him with all his gifts. I said, "Matt, God had to bring you low, because God works in the weak. Now you have to ask for strength to accept it." Amazingly, he agreed. He said, "I hear what you're saying. It's going to be hard, but that's what I have to do."

3

CYNTHIA

AROUND THE SAME TIME that Matt came back from Atlanta, Cynthia, an old friend of his, returned from Haiti, where she had been doing similar work. Though Matt lived in New Meadow Run (his home in Pennsylvania) and Cynthia in Woodcrest (a Bruderhof in New York), they had kept in touch for years.

Cynthia, a feisty young woman, was a little on the wild side. She was also known for her capacity to talk nonstop, to get into heated arguments, and to hold her own when someone stepped on her toes. She was, in other words, a perfect match for Matt.

After high school, Cynthia first tried college, and then a restaurant job at a four-star resort. Neither seemed to click. It was only during a stint in Haiti, where she worked for the national press corps (and later at a hospital), that things began to happen. In her words: "I went to Haiti with very little need for God, my parents, or my friends. I felt like I could handle anything the world could throw at me. I soon found out that I was wrong." She also found out that the rules people played by at home in New York meant nothing in Port-au-Prince, a teeming city that often seemed more like a simmering cauldron of destitution and violence.

After a few months there, Cynthia moved to Cap Haitian, a smaller, less frenetic city. She arrived sick, and found her room crawling with cockroaches. What weighed most on her, however, was a nagging sense of helplessness. She felt directionless and alone. Writing to her parents in November 1997, she said:

> My main problem at the moment is the social life. Wherever I go here I have to run away from men. Everybody wants me because I'm white. There's a girl working at the hospital here whom I like, but her crowd smokes weed and parties all night. Basically I have to say no all the time to everything that comes my way, and I don't think I'll be able to last much longer.
>
> In a country as unstable as this one, where everything is "legal," where you can kill someone for nothing and it is perfectly acceptable, where life is so cheap that stillborn babies are just thrown in the trash, where

bodies are left lying on the side of the road, where only the fit survive, what did I expect would happen to me? That I could just keep on living, and ignore everything I see? I've tried, for a long time. I can feel my emotions going numb, and soon things won't disturb me like they should. Soon I'll be able to walk down the street like everyone else and not even look twice. I'll be able to pay the maid a dollar and not feel any pity for her. I'll even be able to walk into a hospital room and step over a dead body without thinking.

Then came a night that brought everything into focus:

I let myself be dragged along to a rock concert at a hotel where an enormous crowd was celebrating. Around 4:00 a.m. the police began breaking up the party, and a mass of stoned partygoers poured through the lobby where I was waiting to catch my ride home. People were shouting and firing shots into the sidewalk (everyone seems to carry firearms here).

Things quickly got totally out of hand. Guns were going off all over the place, fights were starting, and cars and trucks were jamming the entrance to the hotel. I was really worried. Where was my taxi? I was sure I would get shot, and I started thinking about home, about everything I still wanted to do with my life, about how stupid it was to be stranded where I was. But it was too late.

I started to pray, which felt really strange. I had never needed to pray that hard before, and I wasn't even sure if my prayers would go anywhere. I told God that I wasn't ready to die yet, and that I needed to get out of there, now. Just then, a battered car came screeching up the hill. An old man leaned his head out the window and asked me if I needed a ride. He was high – he appeared to be sniffing glue – but I had no time to be finicky, so I got in. I thought he was an angel…I can still see that car, to this day.

After that incident, things changed:

I'm not sure how or even why, but I began to realize how much I needed God. I actually knew that God was missing from my life all along, but until then I hadn't wanted to admit it. I wanted to see how far I could go on my own. Instead I found myself at the mercy of men, drugs, alcohol, etc.

I also hardened my heart against the suffering I saw. It's not that I wanted to. A lot of things broke me up, and I'd ask, "Why them and not me? Why do some people have to spend their whole life hustling, stealing, and fighting just to stave off hunger each day? Why do some mothers have to give birth to their children in the middle of the street? Why do some two-year-olds, instead of playing in a yard, have to dodge in and out between eight lanes of traffic trying to sell cigarettes?" I wanted to help

them, but knew I couldn't really give them anything. So I looked away and gradually stopped caring. I was unhappy about that, but helpless and
frustrated.

Finally I lost all faith in God. Deep inside, I still
wanted him, but I wasn't ready to get down on my
knees and ask him to help me. Not until that night at
the hotel. After that I knew there was no other help I
could count on – nothing at all, except God's help –
and that's when I decided to start living for him, or
at least for something greater than myself.

By spring 1998, Cynthia was back at Woodcrest. A few
months later Matt's work took him there too. No one
was happier than Cynthia:

Matt was probably my best friend. We spent a lot of
time just talking, playing volleyball, that kind of stuff.
Matt was someone you could talk for hours with;
someone who was willing to discuss real issues. He
was also someone I could get mad or upset at, and
he'd still understand. Later, in early 1999, he moved
back to Pennsylvania, and I remember thinking,
"Why is he leaving, just when we've become best
friends?" I really had to struggle to let go of him.

Matt enjoyed hanging out with Cynthia, but he didn't
see their relationship as anything serious. Confiding
in a close friend shortly before he was diagnosed, he

said, "I'm not interested in getting married. Not this year or next year or three years from now. For one thing, I'm unprepared for such a step; besides, I'm only twenty-two and still have a lot of living to do."

On Thanksgiving weekend, Cynthia heard that Matt had been hospitalized. She was worried but tried not to show it. After all, none of her friends knew how much she cared for him. Later, when she heard that he might have cancer, she fell apart. "I cried for four days. I just couldn't understand why it had to happen to *him*."

On November 30 she wrote him a card:

Matt,

I wanted to write you a short note to wish you a lot of faith in God, knowing that he will do what is best for you. I have asked myself "Why?" many times, and will not ever understand why things like this happen to people, but it has made me turn to God, because it seems that none of us take life seriously enough until it's too late. Don't lose courage, and know that many prayers are being said on your behalf. I believe God will hear them. All that really matters is the relationship each one of us has with him. Keep the faith. God can do anything. Believe that. I wish you the best,

Cynthia

Over the next days Matt e-mailed Christoph several times, sharing new details about his prognosis and grappling with his emotions and the growing role of faith in his personal life. He also solicited a little pastoral advice:

> I can say that Cynthia is really one of *the* best friends I have – and I mean a real friend. She wrote me a letter after she heard that I was sick. I've typed it up for you to read.
>
> I feel that a relationship with Cynthia would be very good for me. It would be a tremendous help in keeping my spirits up. My problem is that I don't know whether it is fair to ask her. I have no question that she would accept if I asked her. But realistically, my chances are not that great, and so it is a very big thing to ask. This is where I need your advice.
>
> If I am not cured, it's no big deal for me, but Cynthia will have to live with it afterwards. I realize that this is just speculation, and that if we both trust in God the right thing will happen in the end, but I had to tell you my reservations. Also, there is no way I want her to do anything out of pity for me.

Replying the same day, Christoph wrote:

> I was touched by the card Cynthia sent to you. Thank you for passing it on. To me it seems quite obvious that she loves you, and that cancer doesn't seem to stand in her way. In regards to your sen-

tence, "If I am not cured…she will have to live with it afterwards," that may be so. But it's not the whole truth. Even in the worst case – if you are married only for one week – it could mean more than a marriage of fifty or sixty years. Trust God, and he will show you the way.

Cynthia, meanwhile, sought advice as well: first from her parents – they were taken aback at first, but then fully supportive – and then from Christoph and his wife. Mostly, however, she kept her thoughts to herself. For one thing, she strongly felt that a friendship with Matt, especially one that led to marriage, could be fruitful only if pursued in accordance with God's will "for my future, and for Matt's." And discerning that would require prayer, not talk. At the same time she found herself growing strangely calm about the matter, despite her unanswered questions: "It was like all my worries and sadness fell away. I felt: if Matt really has to have cancer, he can have cancer. I love him, and if you truly love someone, you love him all the more when he's sick. You don't just think of yourself and what you might lose."

A few days later, Cynthia moved to New Meadow Run to be closer to him. Matt, of course, was overjoyed. So was his mother:

In the days right after Matt came home from the hospital, Randy and I had many tearful discussions.

We were both still very emotional from the sudden shock of Matt's illness, and we wanted so much to support him. How do I keep a positive attitude, I wondered, when all I feel like doing is cry? I worried over whether Matt was at peace with God; whether he was getting enough rest; whether he was getting worn out by too many visitors.

I also worried about marriage – that it would be denied him. To be honest, that was one of the first things that occurred to me after hearing his diagnosis. I remember telling Randy in tears, "I just feel so bad that he will never have anyone to love, like I love you. He won't have anyone to hold him when he's scared, or a foot to touch at night when he can't sleep."

But now Cynthia was there, and Linda could hardly contain her happiness: "Their relationship brought so much joy into that horrible situation." Confessing to Matt how she had worried that he would never have anyone to love, he grinned at his mother and said, "Well, I have someone now."

Cynthia's mother, Gladys, found the development bittersweet at best. Though happy that her daughter was in love, she was also anxious. It wasn't the change taking place in Cynthia – from loud to quiet, from superficial to pensive – that bothered her. She'd expected that. It was her daughter's future as a fiancée and a spouse that she was worried about. "Often I was on the verge of tears," admits Gladys. "Everyone was congratulating me, saying how happy I must be. And I *was* happy. But sometimes I felt like screaming, 'Don't you understand? This isn't just about falling in love! Matt's got cancer; he might be gone within months! How is my daughter going to cope with that?'"

By mid-December, Matt and Cynthia felt that marriage was indeed God's will for them. Three days before Christmas they made their intentions public, requesting (as before every wedding at the Bruderhof) the community's permission and blessing, and receiving both. Two weeks later, on January 9, 2000, they were married.

Throughout the weekend-long wedding festivities, they received one well-wisher after another – hundreds of guests took part – and no one who was there is likely to forget the powerful symbolism of the event. Held as it was in the face of such deep-seated fears, the celebration was an unparalleled affirmation of life, love, and hope.

At the wedding service, portions of a sermon by the nineteenth-century writer J. C. Blumhardt were read. Entitled "Protesters against Death," it had been chosen by Matt and Cynthia because of the striking way in which it expressed the spiritual dimensions of the step they were about to take, and the seriousness of the battle they sensed lay ahead:

> How many people moan and wail when they see that something is mortally wrong with them and that

they must suffer the actual pangs of death. But whatever happens, remember that Jesus also died and came to life. He is with us, and although we must taste death, we know that it does not matter...

If, through tribulation, anxiety, and need, something in you seems to be shattered, let it be shattered. Have no fear, even if you must suffer. Recognize that you are not such a strong person as you thought you were...Remain resolute in seeking the power of eternal life.

Those who try pathetically to push every test away from themselves in the hope that things will go smoothly and easily for them cannot be used in the spiritual fight...

My friends, God does not want to plague you. He wants to use you as a soldier...Therefore turn your difficult days into fighting days. Cry out and pray; look up to heaven, awake, expectant...Then you will be of more use to the kingdom of God than a healthy man. Healthy days often produce little more than a cheerless heart and a dull spirit. Sick days, however, can make us citizens of heaven.

At the end of the ceremony Matt addressed the gathering, his voice brimming with emotion as he spoke:

I just want you all to know that I wouldn't trade my life for anybody else's. If I could go back two months and choose not to have cancer and continue my life

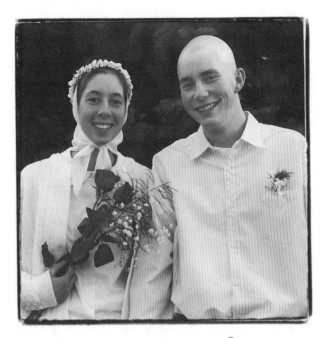

The Wedding Day

as it was, I wouldn't do it. Seriously. I can honestly say that I've never been happier. And it's not just because it's my wedding day. I have felt this ever since I came home from the hospital.

By noon the bride and groom were gone, honeymooning at a nearby cabin. But around 8 p.m. Jonathan's pager went off. It was Matt. As he picked up the phone and dialed the number, Jonathan's mind raced over the last few days. Cynthia had been enthusiastic to learn all she could about Matt's care, and just before the wedding she and Jonathan had gone over everything in his compartmentalized medicine box: frequency, dosage, which tablets belonged where. She had even learned how to administer a Neupogen shot by practicing with a saline-filled syringe. But there was always a chance something could go wrong…

Luckily, there was no need to worry. It was Matt on the line, and he wanted to know whether he could give Cynthia one of his Kytril tablets. After fighting off nausea all afternoon, she had just lost her dinner. "We haven't even been married one day," Matt laughed, "and here *I* am having to care for *her* 'in health and in sickness…'"

4

LIFE WITH CHEMO

MENTION CHEMOTHERAPY, and the first
thing that comes to most people's minds is nausea. It
was certainly the first thing Matt's oncologist thought
of when he described the treatment he was planning:
"Chemo makes the patient sick as a dog. But Matt's
lymphoma will only respond to the most aggressive
protocol we have. He's going to be sick as *three* dogs."

Unbelievably, nothing could have been further
from the truth. There were rough spots during the
initial cycle in December, including feverish nights
and bouts of vomiting. And as the poisons did their
work, killing off cancerous cells (and taking healthy
ones too), Matt began to lose his hair by the handful.
Even so, he generally ate well and kept his food down.
And though he had lost nineteen pounds in late No-

vember and early December, by New Year's Day he was back up to his normal weight.

While jubilant, Matt's oncologists were somewhat mystified. True, he was taking two relatively new medicines that were at least in part responsible for his remarkable progress. One was to counter vomiting; the other to boost white blood cell production. But he was defying *every* expectation, and so quickly...

To Matt, it was simple: though never dismissive of medicine, he felt it was the prayers of those around him that really sustained him. And marriage. As he told Jonathan, "People talk about the benefits of cancer support groups, and the importance of living life as normally as possible. But there's really no better support group than a wife!" Cynthia agreed. Writing to a friend shortly after Christmas, she elated:

> It is overwhelming how Matt is doing – so well that it's hard to believe he still has cancer. Now we need to thank God...and to hope for other individuals who need healing. It *can* happen. We have never been so happy and thankful to be alive...We love each other a lot, and want to use our love for God, not ourselves. We have confidence in everything.

Life wasn't all roses, however, and if some days passed with smiles, others dragged on with depressing conversations and the re-emergence of old fears. Sometimes the questions seemed to come out of the blue – though for Matt, they were surely always there, lurking in the back of his mind.

"I don't think we've talked about outcome yet, have we, Jonathan?" he asked one day.

"Actually, we have, Matt. Nothing's changed. Statistically, you still have a fifty percent chance of surviving five years. But that really doesn't mean much."

Matt seemed surprised. "That's not very good," he mused, staring off into space.

At other times, discussions about the future were more philosophical, as Matt weighed up the value of knowing one's statistical prognosis or considered the reminder – by a staff person at the hospital – that chemo would interfere with his chances of ever being a father. Yes, he'd thought about the "fertility issue," but at the time he'd been desperate simply to stay alive. As he told Jonathan, "There are so many big ifs to worry about at once." (Understandably, the question of parenthood gained new importance – and caused no little amount of heartache – after Matt and Cynthia's wedding in January.)

If having children of their own was impossible, though, there were still plenty of others around to cheer them up. Like every apartment at the Bruderhof, Matt and Cynthia's was part of a larger multi-family unit, and if Jonathan's children didn't invite themselves down for a story or a board game (the family lived in the same split-level house), Matt would be sure to invite one himself.

Matt's love of children extended to the community school – he had taught a boy's gym class the previous year – and even when he could no longer shoot hoops with them, he still made an effort to stay involved. Near the end of January, the editors of the school magazine requested an interview, asking Matt to describe his illness and wanting to know the impact it had on his plans for the future.

Matt obliged, but only halfway. "Please make your magazine funnier," he wrote to the young reporter who wanted to talk with him, "and don't ask silly questions like about me being sick." In the end, the interview proceeded, but only after Matt was promised a new topic – sports:

1. What do you think about pro sports in general (salaries, etc.)?

2. Does following pro sports take your mind off your sickness?

3. What are your favorite teams, and why do you like them?"

Matt responded:

1. Pro sports in general? That's kind of a tough question, because there are pros and cons…As far as salaries go – yeah, the players are overpaid, but

people want to see them play, and so will shell out $40 to go see ten guys run around for less than an hour. It's a distraction, like all entertainment, and gives people a break from their own boring lives. They used to say that religion was the opiate of the people, but nowadays it's entertainment, with professional sports being right up there at the top of the list of culprits. But I like them anyway and certainly wouldn't want to see them go. Hey, if you could go shoot hoops for $33 million a year, wouldn't you?

2. I told you not to ask me about that, so you don't get an answer to this question.

3. My favorite teams are all from Minnesota, which is where I grew up. They include the Vikings (football), Twins (baseball), and Golden Gophers (college). Notice that I have always liked these teams and am not a fair-weather fan like all these jokers who all of a sudden like the Yanks or the Rams just because they are doing well…The sign of a true fan is someone who sticks with his team through thick and thin.

Throughout Matt's illness, the community that surrounded him and Cynthia provided them with an all-encompassing net of safety and support. It was seldom that Matt went unmentioned in the community's regular evening meetings, and when the going was especially rough, it was not unusual for a peer, nurse, or neighbor to call a quiet, impromptu vigil besides. Given that the Bruderhof has members in the United States, England, and Australia, there must have been many days when Matt was prayed for literally around the clock.

In addition, Randy and Linda's work schedules were rearranged to allow them as much time as they wanted with their son, and after the wedding, Cynthia's family was provided with an apartment near her and Matt, and invited to stay on as long as they wanted. "I can't imagine our experience outside of a community of people who love and care for one another," Randy reflected later. "Linda and I were basically relieved of all our work-related responsibilities for six months. Where else can you find that?"

Moreover, if the community's adult members ever slackened in their intercession, they were reminded of that duty by their children. Jonathan recalls an evening around Christmas:

> I was tucking my children in, and one of them wanted to pray for Matt. First he told me that he was going to pray kneeling with his hands clasped, which he did, and then he knelt with upturned hands as well. After that he climbed into bed, but then jumped out again suddenly and said that he also wanted to pray for Matt standing up, with his arms spread wide. "I have seen that kind of praying in books," he told me. And

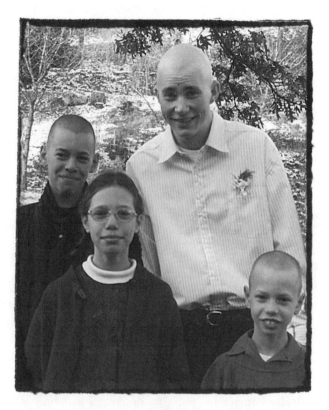

With Jonathan's kids

how could God *not* hear such intense, triplicate prayers?

Still, Matt remained anxious about the particulars of his chemo throughout each of its six scheduled cycles. Though well aware of his need for prayer, and conscious of the importance of a positive outlook, part of him clung desperately to the physiological ins and outs of the regimen – as if a precise knowledge of what was happening to his body would somehow better his odds. He was especially nervous, for instance, about his rescue medication – drugs used to counteract the powerful toxins injected during chemo – and when they arrived from the pharmacy he insisted on knowing exactly where they were and fretted about whether it was the safest place. Happily, Cynthia's companionship relaxed him tremendously, so much so that before receiving his second round of injections, in January, he split a bag of Doritos with her while sitting in the waiting room.

Meeting other people with cancer helped Matt look beyond his illness, too, especially when he realized how lonely some of them were. Cynthia usually had to coax him to engage someone in conversation, but she says he always admitted afterward that reaching out to someone in the waiting room could make the most depressing trip at least a little brighter. One time they met a patient who promised she'd go out that evening and drum to the moon for Matt. "That's the way I talk to God," she explained. Tossing and turning all that night, Matt muttered the next morning that "that kind of prayer" must not work too well.

Remembering Matt's trips to the hospital, Linda still laughs about the shirt he insisted on wearing almost every time – a tattered, gray knit he'd picked up while working at a clothing bank for the homeless in Atlanta:

> It shrank once in the machine, and he would never let me touch it after that. He loved that shirt so much that he insisted on washing it by hand. After he got sick, he wore it more often. I don't know why. Perhaps it was cozy or just made him feel normal or himself.
>
> Anyway, whenever he had to go to chemo, he'd come out of his room wearing it, and I'd encourage him to put on something dressier – anything but that shirt. But he'd give me this little twinkle and say, "It's my homeless shirt, Mom. It's important to identify with the homeless." And that's just how it made him look – homeless.

Then there was Vern – a stuffed camel that arrived from Henry, Matt's old high school bosom buddy, shortly after he got sick. Cynthia remembers:

> It had a really dumb face and curly hair. It was supposed to look after Matt and help him feel better.

Matt loved it and kept it by his bed at all times, partly because he thought about Henry a lot. When I came into the picture, we found a name for this camel. We called it Vern after the guy in the movie *Rain Man*.

Matt was so attached to this camel. I had never gotten that emotional with stuffed animals myself. I would walk into the bedroom and find Matt asleep, holding Vern. Pretty soon, Vern became a joke between us, and I would hide him – though always where I knew Matt would eventually find him. Sometimes it took him a couple days, and then he'd hide Vern from me. Soon we had a contest going over who could hide him in the best place. Vern landed up in the bathroom, the shower, the medicine cabinet, the dresser, the bed, the pillow cases, hanging from the ceiling, shoes – everywhere you can think of.

Once, Matt hid Vern in his jacket and brought him along on a walk. He tried to distract me, and then, when I wasn't watching him, he quickly threw Vern so he would land on the road in front of us. Unfortunately, Vern landed in a ditch, so there was nothing to see when I turned around. Matt didn't know what to do at first, and for a minute I thought he was losing it – he looked so surprised. Then he started laughing, and told me to look in the ditch. There was Vern, all dirty and rejected-looking, with his stupid face staring up at us. I've never laughed so hard – not at Vern, but because Matt had gone to such lengths to outdo me in hiding a stuffed animal.

I had to get back at him. The next day, when Matt was in the shower, I took his underwear and put it on Vern. Matt took a really long time getting dressed. When he finally came out, he saw Vern and just about collapsed laughing. This sort of thing went on even during the last weeks of Matt's life, when he was really sick. Vern was always by his bedside.

I never would have thought that something so simple could make two adults so happy. But when you have cancer, you have to be stupid sometimes. At least Matt and I did. We laughed and joked and sometimes made so much noise that the neighbors who lived in the next apartment came running down the hall to see what the hell was going on.

Matt's golf cart, which he used to get to events around the community, was another source of laughs, Cynthia says:

> When other people were around, Matt drove slowly and courteously. But once they were out of sight, he'd hit the gas, and we went around most corners on two wheels. I think I have a permanent bruise on my right hip from being slammed against the side rail.
>
> One time we were driving along a path, and smack in the middle of the road was this huge, black

pot-bellied pig tied to a rope. It was Alice, a neighbor's pet. Matt stepped on the gas and headed
straight toward Alice, certain she would move out
of the way. But she didn't. We were only a few feet
away when he realized that if he didn't slam on the
brakes *now,* there'd be BLT's for dinner. We came
within inches of her nose.

In general, Matt's progress throughout the winter was
so steady that at times he forgot all about having cancer – or so he gloated at a routine medical check-up
one day. Jonathan replied, "That's great – you should
do that more often!" at which Matt unexpectedly
burst into tears: "Yeah, but the bad part is suddenly
remembering it again. Then everything comes to a
halt, and you find yourself gulping with the heaviness
of it all." Jonathan reminded him that his future was
in God's hands and encouraged him to trust in that.
But Matt would not be consoled.

As Cynthia later put it, "Having cancer is like living on a yo-yo. One day you're jerked up, and the next
day you're dropped." If there was anything constant,
she says, it was the regularity with which Matt worried
about a recurrence. On the one hand, he could not
have been happier with the way things were going, especially in mid-February, when they traveled to New
York and spent several days at Woodcrest. On the other
hand, he never forgot the speed with which the cancer

had attacked him in November, nor the doctors' pre-
diction at the time: if it ever came back, there'd be little
they could do. Cynthia says:

> Because of this, the smallest cold threw us for a loop,
> which was totally distressing – to think that, for the
> rest of his life, every little thing could make him
> doubt his health. He said, "I don't want to be scared
> forever."
>
> On the other hand, he insisted that he wasn't
> afraid to die. He told me, "What's hard is the idea of
> letting go of all the little things that life is made of –
> going to work, seeing kids outside playing ball, just
> being with other people. Things I've always taken for
> granted. I used to think that when people get cancer,
> the thing they fear most is death. Now I think the
> biggest thing is disappointment. It's realizing your
> life will never be the same again."

Nevertheless, such recognitions deepened Matt and
Cynthia's love for one another more than anything
else in their marriage. Recounting an especially significant conversation that took place one night in
February, Cynthia says:

> We had come home from an evening meeting where
> there'd been a very thought-provoking discussion
> about what it means to live for the kingdom of God,
> and after we stayed up a little, we put the lights out
> and went to bed. Suddenly Matt said, "I was just

thinking about something." I asked him, "What?" He was quiet for a moment, and then said, "Oh, forget it. I can't tell you, because it will make you scared." First I thought it had something to do with his sickness, so I was tempted to leave it at that, but then I got curious and convinced him to tell me what was up. He said, "Well, you know, I was thinking about how soon I might be seeing the kingdom." He was really excited by that thought.

I had never thought about the future like that, and I was scared. What scared me, I guess, was the thought that everything will come to an end, and we will all have to die. But then we talked about it some, and I realized that I was thinking of myself and everything I enjoy in life, and not about God, and I kind of lost it and started crying.

Matt felt really bad, because he thought he'd upset me. But I told him I wasn't crying because I was sad. I was crying because now I was also excited, and wanted to go to the kingdom too. As far as I was concerned, I wanted it to come right then and there, so that we could go together. I guess it had finally hit me that God's kingdom is the answer for all the suffering people in the world, and that it's not going to come until we pray for it to happen.

In spite of such sobering moments, though, it was impossible for either Matt or Cynthia to ignore his continued improvement. Why should they? On

March 27, his white count was the highest it had been for months, and on March 28, he received his long-awaited final round of chemo. ("You're all done, Matt!" proclaimed a child's welcome sign on the front door back at home. "Just say no to drugs!" said another.)

On March 30, he had his hospital bed removed – a sign of better times coming, he said – and sent an e-mail to Christoph, telling him that his treatments were finally over, and that he was doing fine. Jonathan, however, wrote in his journal that same night that he felt the battle was "far from over." And he couldn't help thinking of a comment his four-year-old had made at bedtime: "Daddy, we still need to pray for Matt."

5

BACK TO THE FRONT

APRIL STARTED OUT as happily as March had ended. Matt's hair began to grow back in, he exercised daily, and most important to him, he resumed work with a regularity he hadn't been able to maintain since the previous November. Some days he did programming for the community publishing house, where among other things he logged onto a co-worker's computer and sent prank e-mails; other days he surprised the "shop brothers" at the community's furniture factory by showing up there.

In the middle of the month his parents returned to Australia, where their absence from the new community had slowed work on several fronts, and at a send-off celebration held the night before they went, they talked about meeting there by summer's end.

But that was not to be. If anything, Randy and Linda's departure marked the beginning of a long slide downhill. From Jonathan's journal:

April 16: Matt has been increasingly fatigued, with aching joints, headaches, and a productive cough for several days…His lungs are fine, though, and he has no backache. It seems to be just a typical viral infection, perhaps with some additional arthralgias. I don't feel it is anything connected to his malignancy, and I have reassured him about this, although of course we never really know.

April 24 : Cynthia called to let me know how nervous Matt is about tomorrow – his first exam since chemo. I know it's a milestone of sorts, but the blood work is routine, and then it's just the usual twenty to thirty questions, and an external check for nodes. Yet she says he's had a couple good cries about it already, and told her that he "won't be surprised if Jonathan finds something." Apparently she admonished him and said he should have more faith that everything will go well. He replied that they ought to be prepared, just in case it *doesn't.*

Matt's partly right, of course, and I told Cynthia that perhaps he is just steeling himself against bad news. And yet, we do not have any bad news at this time, and need to keep our spirits up and remain strong. I realize again how fragile we all are, and how easily medical questions can distract us from what is

truly important. Everything needs to be kept in the
right perspective…

April 25: Met with Matt this morning…We discussed
sleep, appetite, energy, weight, skin, cough, hypersen-
sitive fingertips, etc., at length. The examination was
entirely negative except for a rash on his legs. No
nodes palpated at all. Matt clearly keyed up, but reassured that all is well, at least externally…I broke the
news to him about the bone marrow aspirate on May
15, and he is not happy. He asked me twice whether it
will be as bad as the last one…We also went over
other upcoming appointments and tests.

May 3: Matt is completely off his sleeping medications now. We'll see how things go.

On May 6, Roland, an elderly family friend whom
Matt knew well, passed away unexpectedly and
peacefully in his sleep. Matt was deeply shaken when
he heard the news, and went to his room and cried.
"He just fell apart," Cynthia told Jonathan later that
day. "He would like to die like Roland, suddenly and
painlessly, but he doesn't think he will. He's really
scared. He knows he is going to suffer." To Cynthia, it
was as if Roland's death heralded Matt's:

Every day when I woke up, I would ask him, "How
are you feeling?" I wanted so badly to hear him say
that he was feeling better, but each day was either the

same as the day before, or worse. We would just lie there and cry, and pray to God to please help us. We were constantly being forced onto our knees.

The thought of the upcoming tests was almost unbearable. Right before the first one, Matt had high fevers and started vomiting so violently, I can still hear him retching when I think about it. I tried to be strong for him, and told him everything was going to be all right, but inside I was so scared. I needed someone to tell *me* that everything would be all right. I would sit there next to him and pray and pray and pray: "God, make it stop." I felt so helpless. Matt would shake his head and say, "There's something wrong. They need to find out what it is now." But then always he'd try to be strong, because he knew how hard it was for me to watch him and not be able to help.

On Mother's Day, May 14, Matt woke up feeling really nauseated. He sat on the edge of our bed and retched like he'd been doing for the past two weeks. It was heartbreaking. I stepped into the bathroom for a few minutes, and when I came out, there on the dresser was the most gorgeous bouquet I'd ever seen: twenty-four red roses! Matt was still sitting on the bed, bucket in hand, but he gave me his winning smile and said, "Happy Mother's Day." That was how Matt loved me. He would do anything, no matter how sick he was…

Two days later, on May 16, Matt went in to Morgantown, where a CT scan and chest x-ray revealed
pneumonia and slightly enlarged nodes in the chest.
The oncologist was certain that the nodes were enlarged because of the pneumonia, not malignancy,
but his optimism did little to calm anyone's nerves.
As Cynthia remembers it:

> Our fear was indescribable. Walking down the hospi-
> tal halls, Matt went into nearly every bathroom we
> passed because he had to throw up. I would wait out-
> side, my head as close to the door as possible, so I
> could hear if he was all right. Then I got sick, too,
> from the stress. So there we were, both vomiting. It
> was a nightmare.
>
> At one point, we just started crying. Matt got
> really frustrated and said, "I've had enough! I can't
> take it anymore!" I felt exactly the same. I was fall-
> ing apart emotionally and had had all I could take.
> I needed comfort and reassurance myself, and real-
> ized that there was no way I could support Matt
> like I wanted to right then. I must have cried all
> the way home from the hospital.

That evening the entire community, including many
of the children, met to intercede for Matt. "We were
grateful for their support, but neither of us went,"
says Cynthia. "We just stayed home and cried."

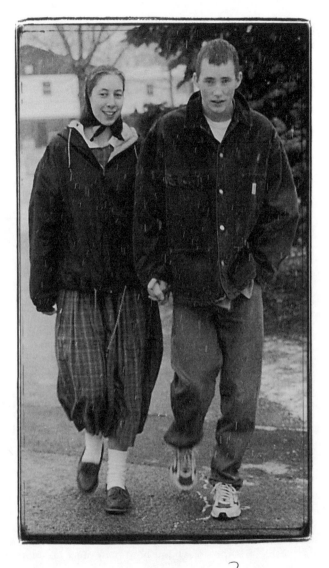

Where's Vern?

The next morning Matt returned to Morgantown for a PET scan to double-check his enlarged nodes for evidence of cancer. The results were reassuring. Jonathan wept silent tears of thanks, but had cold feet, noting that "the best PET scan is imprecise," and reminding Matt and Cynthia that the cancer could still return at any time. Back at home, however, word that Matt was "in remission" spread like wildfire and swept up the entire community in a celebratory mood.

Looking back on those days, Cynthia says they were probably the most difficult she ever endured. One moment she radiated over Matt's "healing"; the next, she found herself filled with a strange dread.

> Of course we were happy about the PET scan. But Matt wasn't feeling any better, and when you aren't feeling well, and haven't been for over a month, you want to know what's wrong with you. We were so frustrated. Our minds were telling us one thing – "it can't be the cancer" – and our guts another – "it's back." We didn't know what to feel or think. Were we lacking in faith because we were scared deep down inside? Were we lacking in faith because we doubted the medical results? Were we lacking in faith because Matt was dying? What is faith, anyway? Deep down we felt that it meant trusting in God's will, no matter what. But you don't know how many times I tried to convince myself that it simply meant praying more, and believing that Matt would be cured.

Jonathan, too, yearned to affirm the optimistic outlook of other community members, but worried in
his journal that "we weak human beings sure place a
lot of trust in medical tests – too much." After all,
Matt was worsening, not improving. Still, he argued
with himself, who but a pessimist would ignore good
news?

Early on the morning of May 24, Jonathan, who
was in Lexington, Kentucky, attending a medical
conference, received a phone call. It was Matt. He
said he had a fever of over 105° F and was feeling
lots of painful nodes, both in his groin and else-
where. Jonathan listened, mumbled some words of
comfort, and numbly hung up. Afterwards, too dis-
tracted to attend the day's lectures, he went to a
quiet park, stared at the fountains, and immersed
himself in prayer. "What else could I do?" he remembers asking himself. Around noon, however, he
called a colleague at home and asked her to arrange
for one of Matt's enlarged nodes to be biopsied. "I
don't trust the PET scan at all," he told her. He also
decided to leave the conference a day early.

Driving home the next day Jonathan couldn't
help thinking of Adela, an old classmate who had
been diagnosed with Hodgkin's lymphoma several
years earlier. At that time the community had prayed
ardently for healing, and many, including Adela's

fiancé (who married her despite her cancer) were hopeful. After all, the doctors had given her an eighty-five percent chance of survival. Yet a few years later Adela had died, becoming, as her grief-stricken father, Jacob, later put it, "one of the other fifteen percent." What lay in store for Matt?

By late afternoon the next day, Matt was lying on an operating table in Morgantown with Jonathan at his side, while Cynthia and her parents waited nearby. Jacob and his wife, who had come along to provide additional support, sat with them.

The surgeon worked speedily, removing two almond-sized nodes from the right side of Matt's neck and sending them immediately to the pathologist on call. Within minutes the incision was sutured, and an orderly prepared to wheel Matt out of the room. Just then the pathologist called back. She had found malignant cells, "almost identical to the lymphoma found last December." Jonathan gulped and bit his lip. His legs went weak. Everyone was silent.

Cynthia broke down when the surgeon came out and told her the news: "But God has answered our prayers so wonderfully this far, and now this!" Comforting her as best he could, Jacob gently reminded Cynthia that while he understood her disbelief perfectly, she must remember that "our lives are in God's hands at all times," and further, that "our constant prayer has been, Thy will be done."

Back in the recovery room, Matt was slowly waking up. Jonathan went to get Cynthia, and when they returned Matt was awake. Cynthia took both of his hands and whispered into his ear, "It's back. The cancer is back." Matt stared blankly for a moment, then blurted, "Let's get out of here! Can't we go to a quiet room? I need to think!"

At home, the community was meeting for evening worship, and when Christoph, who had just talked with Jonathan, reported on Matt's condition, many burst into tears. Pointing out that Matt's life was now drawing to a close, Christoph went on to ponder the meaning of true healing, and noted that while people often pray for physical healing, it is spiritual healing that is of utmost importance. He also pointed out that although Matt might seem young, there is no such thing as an "untimely" death, for as the Bible says, "to God, a thousand years are like one day." At the end of the meeting, someone suggested setting up a vigil room where different ones could come at any hour of the day or night to pray, sing, or simply contemplate in silence. (Such a room was later prepared, and it was soon in constant use, drawing not only Matt's peers, but also families with children and the elderly.)

Meanwhile Matt's parents were sitting at the airport in Sydney, gearing up – for the second time in six months – for a long flight home, though dreading the news of what awaited them there. In Randy's words:

Again, we had to wait for hours, and we spent the time looking for little things to bring back for Matt and Cynthia. We picked out some music and then went to a National Geographic store where we found some window stick-ons: parrots and koalas. Linda cried when she realized that all we could get for him was stuff he could look at from his bed. It was so hard to believe that this was happening.

Later I called Steve, our pastor back at home in Pennsylvania. Steve said the news wasn't good; that the cancer was back again, and in many nodes…His voice was shaky, and then he totally broke down. I was numb – unable to say anything except good-bye. For several minutes I couldn't return to Linda. Finally I went back to her. When she turned and looked at me, I simply shook my head, and we both dissolved into tears. Deep inside, both of us knew the outcome of the tests already…

The next morning, Cynthia, worrying that Matt had not yet taken in the gravity of the situation, asked Jonathan to speak with him, "before all the doctors come traipsing through." They discussed the importance of reminding Matt what his oncologists had said all along – that if the cancer came back, there would be nothing to do – and agreed that for Matt's sake, the best thing would surely be to get him home as soon as possible. Cynthia also asked Jonathan to tell Matt "that he needs to be prepared to die soon." Jonathan assured her that he would be open, as always, but added that he felt it would be vital for Matt to sense, first and foremost, their love and caring, and through that "come to this important conclusion himself." As recounted in his journal entry for May 27:

> We went in, and I started by reminding Matt that although we had been praying for physical recovery over these past months, it seemed that the time had now come when we needed to look beyond that. I reminded him that it is the spiritual that is eternal, not the physical, and that even as a doctor I felt that the readiness to accept God's will in one's life is much more important than physical health. I then added, "This readiness may include giving up our physical life."
>
> Matt had been holding Cynthia's hand up till then, but at this he sat bolt upright, grabbed me with his other arm, and looked us straight in the eye, stunned. "You mean I need to be prepared to die – *now?*" "Yes," we answered in unison. It was silent in the room. We then reminded him that our prayers – and the prayers of all our brothers and sisters at home – would carry him through everything, and that what we needed to focus on now was finding strength and courage, and most of all, inner peace.
>
> As he grappled with all this, he had one question after the other, each of which Cynthia tried to answer as straightforwardly as she could. At one

point, as he dissolved in tears, she grabbed his leg and said with great intensity, "But Matt, we have to make every day count! And we have to love each other more. You yourself told me a few months ago that you might be privileged to see the kingdom of God before the end of this year, and you were so excited! You were looking forward to it. We have to find that joy again."

Matt reassured us that he wasn't hanging onto any impossible dreams; he had definitely rejected the idea of a bone marrow transplant, for example, and experimental chemo. But he still wished he could do *something* to "buy me a little more time." Later, however, he rejected every option except palliative care, which we could give him at home, and insisted on leaving the hospital that afternoon.

We left around 3:00 and drove all the way home in complete silence. Once we got there, around 4:00, Cynthia went to bed. Matt was exhausted, too, but told me he was afraid to go to sleep, "because I might stop breathing." After I promised I would stay with him, however, he relaxed somewhat. Holding tight to my hand, he fell asleep within ten or fifteen minutes.

Around 6 p.m. he got up and went into the living room for dinner, after which he sat in his armchair, fed his tropical fish, and chatted with my sons, who had come downstairs to visit. He soon tired, and I decided to take the boys home. As we left he called weakly after us, "You guys come down again real soon, okay? I'm going to need you now, more than ever."

Hours later, too anxious to sleep, Matt was still sitting in his armchair, waiting for his parents to arrive from the airport. They got in around 1 a.m. Cynthia recalls:

> I looked out the window and saw people standing outside, lining the path and holding lanterns and torches. I told Matt to come look. His parents were walking up to the house, and the whole community had started singing. We stood in the dark room, watching them – we were holding each other and sobbing – and we stayed there till Matt's parents walked in the door.

Once inside the house, there were long, tearful embraces. Matt settled into an armchair, with Randy right next to him, and Cynthia and Linda curled up on the couch. No one knew what to say. Finally Matt phoned Jonathan and asked him if he could come down and give his parents a quick rundown of the previous weeks. As Randy wrote in his diary:

> Bone marrow transplant is out, and aside from that, there is nothing else to do for this kind of cancer at this point. Matt and Cynthia talk of being ready for further chemo if it will help. I have doubts in my mind, but now is not the time to bring them up. None of us want him to die. His cough is terrible…

Silence followed, after which Randy reminded Matt that many people on this earth face death alone, without any support or love. "We have each other," he said, "and we can love each other every day that you have left." He then added that everyone has to face death sometime, and told Matt, "You are just going ahead of us." Linda, who had left the couch, was embracing her son: "I told him over and over, 'I'm *so* sorry!' either out loud or to myself – I couldn't say. As a mom, all you want to do when your child is sick is make things better. But I couldn't, and so I said I was sorry."

6

LEARNING TO LET GO

TWO DAYS after Matt learned that his cancer had returned, he e-mailed Christoph, sharing his relief at being home, and commenting on his feeling that his life was no longer in human hands: "Just wanted to let you know that I am home, and very happy about that…They were planning to do one more procedure in the hospital yesterday afternoon, but I told them to forget it. You can only do so much and then you just have to quit and leave the rest to God."

The following day he reiterated the same thought to a friend who stopped by and told him that he was still "praying for a miracle." Matt replied, "Thanks, but I think it's past that stage. The main thing now is that I find peace."

While such an attitude might have signaled res-
ignation to someone who didn't know Matt, those
close to him knew it was the hard-won fruit of a determined struggle. Over the next three days, Matt
floundered in a sea of warring emotions. Part of
him was so battle-weary that he must have longed,
at times, to close his eyes and go. Another clung desperately to the unlikely prospects of the only remaining medical option, a dose-intensive protocol
with a ninety percent mortality rate.

Linda, too, felt jostled by conflicting waves of
anxiety and hope, and found strength to go on only
through constant prayer. A passage from Macdonald's
Sir Gibbie, in which he describes a woman who "held
the gate open in prayer" for a son lost on the moors,
somehow captured her pain in a particular way, and
she turned to it often:

> "Oh Lord," she said, in her great trusting heart, "If
> my bonnie man be drowning in the water or dying
> of cold on the hillside, hold his hand. Be not far
> from him. O Lord, don't let him be afraid."

Meanwhile, certain members of the community
seemed to act as if Matt's re-diagnosis was simply a
bad dream, and continued to clutch at every piece of
potentially good news. A day or so after Matt returned
from the hospital, a young man cheerfully reassured
Randy, "Matt's *going* to pull out of this!" And a few

days after that a well-meaning neighbor told Linda
that her teenage daughter had said, "Matt is not going
to die. I know he's not going to die."

As Jacob reflected, the tendency to grasp at straws
is a persistent one. "Even when we think we are praying for God's will to be done," he noted, "our actions
sometimes show that we regard prayer as some sort
of vending machine – put in enough, and you'll get
out what you want." Going on, he added:

> Even when it had become obvious that Matt's cancer
> was returning, his doctors were hedging: "It's flu; it's
> pneumonia." But what I heard and saw reminded me
> so much of my daughter's last days. At such times
> there is a strong temptation to avoid the harshness
> of the situation by giving it different names. One
> specialist said that Matt's symptoms were typical of
> tuberculosis. I said, "Give me a break." Technically,
> I'm sure he was right. But I also felt we were missing
> the bigger picture; we were wearing blinders that
> prevented us from seeing what was staring us in the
> face. We weren't allowing ourselves to step back and
> ask, "What does all of this actually mean?" And be-
> cause of this, I think we blocked God from speaking
> to us and stood in his way.

Randy and Linda shared Jacob's concern. For one
thing, they sensed a weakening of Matt's earlier certainty that his life was wholly in God's hands; for

another, they felt that an element of denial had begun
to cloud the clarity of the situation – the obvious fact
that Matt was going to die. On the morning of May
31, they decided to speak up. Linda later recon-
structed their conversation:

> *Randy:* Hey, Matt, we're only concerned that you
> don't hang on to the idea of medical treatments.
> They failed you before; you aren't as strong as you
> were; and they'll be a lot rougher on you this time
> around. They might even kill you.

> *Matt:* But I'm excited about taking more treatments.
> They helped me before. I know they won't cure any-
> thing, but still…I know we have to take one day at a
> time. That's all I'm trying to do. If there is *anything*
> that can help, I want to try it. We can't just give up.

> *Linda:* We agree with you about taking one day at a
> time. We are one-hundred percent with you. We're
> not giving up hope, but we just don't want you to
> hang onto any false hopes, that's all.

> *Randy:* You and Cynthia are the only ones that can
> make the decision about more treatments. We'll be
> with you no matter what you decide, but honestly –
> we'd hate to see you put your hope in further treat-
> ments. The only thing we hope in is God. He will be
> with us.

> *Matt:* Yes, I know…But I also have to keep fighting.

After Matt left the room, Randy and Linda continued to grapple on their own. "It's impossible to convey the emotions of that morning," Randy said later. "We were on the verge of breaking down. Matt was tearful and extremely fragile, and so were we. Physically, he was being propped up by steroids and painkillers that masked his true condition. Emotionally, he was hanging on to a medical "option" that no one – not even his doctors – really believed could help."

What could they do? Finally, they called Jonathan and asked him if they could come over to his office to talk. As Linda said later, "Matt wasn't facing things, but I didn't think he was the only one."

Randy was the first to speak. "I laid it out as straight as we saw it," he recalls. "I said, 'Matt is dying; Matt is terminal. We have to use these words. He is *terminal!*'" Linda went on to say that while she was thankful for all that had been done for Matt so far, she nevertheless felt that further medical intervention of any kind would only make the end much worse.

Jonathan was grateful for the exchange. As he later admitted, "I had to recognize that ultimately, even a simple thing like obliging Matt's request for another chest x-ray or antibiotic was a hindrance, because it would continue to feed a false sense of security and divert him and Cynthia from the fact that he was dying."

"It was so hard," Randy says, "to finally let go after fighting all those months, and to say: I can't do any more. And further, to admit that what I *am* doing is only preventing him from facing death and finding peace. We'd been focused on fighting the disease for six months, and now that focus had to change."

"It was a battle," Linda agrees, "but we were actually in the same boat. We had all prayed for physical healing, all hoped that medicine would help. And when it didn't, our first reaction was to see it as a defeat."

Reliving that strenuous morning, Linda remembered two other similar occasions – both of them equally intense, and equally vital. The first had come one night the previous December, just a few weeks after Matt's initial diagnosis:

> I was in the bathroom, on my knees, crying and praying and struggling. It went on until midnight. I was feeling very possessive and trying to shield Matt from anything that would take him from me. I said to myself that even if it was God's plan for Matt to die, I still wouldn't accept it. I was fighting against God, plain and simple. Finally I was able to confess this to him and to plead for his forgiveness, and later I experienced a deep peace.
>
> Afterward, I asked Randy for forgiveness, too, because I'd been making it very hard for him, and he

didn't know what to do for me. But I guess I just had to fight it out alone. Boy, it was hard! But I realized that true prayer is always hard. Fighting to accept God's will is *fighting* – it means being part of an army – and I had just decided to go AWOL. I was very ashamed that I had such little strength.

Shortly before New Year's, Linda went through round two:

By now I had come to peace about Matt's cancer and felt able to let go of his physical well-being. But then he got engaged, and I suddenly realized how hard it was going to be to give Matt to another woman. What a mix of emotions – "Matt won't need me anymore like he has all these years. I won't be number one on the list of women he loves." On the one hand, I knew his love for Cynthia was such a wonderful gift. On the other hand, I still couldn't give him up completely.

A few years earlier, when Matt had been in Atlanta, I had also struggled with letting him go. I knew that my worrying wouldn't bring him back, and that his life was out of my hands – even though I really wanted it in my hands! I remember telling God that he could have Matt, that Matt was his anyway, and that I couldn't do a thing. But now Matt had cancer and was going to get married, and it all came flooding back. "I want my son back," I told

God. "I didn't really mean it when I said you could have him."

It took all I had to get over that one. I was fighting myself, I was fighting God, I was fighting the devil – I don't know who I was fighting with – but in the end, I *did* give Matt to God again.

But now it was others who were battling, and Linda could not keep silent. Thankfully, the breakthrough came quickly, in a conversation later the same morning. Christoph and his wife, Verena, had come out to Pennsylvania especially to see Matt and Cynthia, and at one point, while sitting with them and discussing the uncertainty of the future, Christoph brought up the very same issue that Matt's parents had brought up just a few hours before:

> You know, Matt, I think the central question here is whether you are ready to die – tomorrow. If you are really ready to go, and Cynthia is ready to let you go, then all other questions, including those about chemotherapy, become peripheral. God can, of course, suddenly reverse things and provide a miracle, but I personally do not think that will happen, and we cannot count on it. Perhaps God has something else in mind for you. It is painful, I know…

Turning to Matt, Christoph said, "Matt, you are dying. Are you ready to die?" And then to Cynthia, "Are you ready to let him go?" The questions hung for a moment. "Something very important – something awesome – is at stake here," he went on. "It is something way bigger than the two of you – way beyond any of us. It is a spiritual matter." There was another silence. Then Cynthia spoke:

> You know, I think we've lost what we felt in the beginning, six months ago: the willingness to give each other up. I think we've clung so much to medicine that we've forgotten the way we used to look forward to God's kingdom. We have to find it again.
>
> I thought I'd fought through letting Matt go before our wedding. But now I'm having to fight it through again. I may be clinging to medicine, but it's not because I'm unwilling to let Matt go. I think it's because I can't face the suffering he might have to go through.

Christoph looked at Matt and Cynthia. "You *are* going to suffer," he said. He then looked at Randy and Linda, who were also in the room. "You are also going to suffer. There's no way around it." Looking back at Matt and Cynthia, he concluded, "It is vital that you two find peace about all this. Whatever you decide, we will support you. Cynthia, it will be terribly hard. Matt *is* going to suffer; both of you will. But I believe it will bring you closer to each other, and closer to God."

Christoph then led the small gathering in prayer, asking God for courage and strength to sustain them in the days ahead. Afterward, in their room, Matt and Cynthia struggled on alone. In Cynthia's words:

> Everyone else left the house for lunch, but Matt and I stayed. We knew we had to decide right then and there what we were going to do. It was not as if Christoph has actually said anything new. Deep down, we'd felt the same. But it was only in that conversation that it finally hit home: we hadn't really been ready to face death and to accept God's will.
>
> Then Matt looked at me and said, "You decide. I'll do whatever you think is best." I told him I couldn't do that; we had to decide together.
>
> Everything in me wanted to take that one last chance with further chemo. Even if it wouldn't work, it might possibly buy us more time. That was all I wanted: time, time, time – time to love each other more...
>
> Yet I couldn't suppress the nagging questions in the back of my mind: What if it worked, and gave us more time, but we weren't supposed to have that time? What if it didn't work, and gave Matt less time than God wanted him to have? Finally, I told Matt that I firmly believed we should leave *everything* to God, and that he would give us whatever time Matt was meant to have. Matt said he felt exactly the same.
>
> Up to that point, he'd seen the idea of declining further treatment as defeat. He'd said many times:

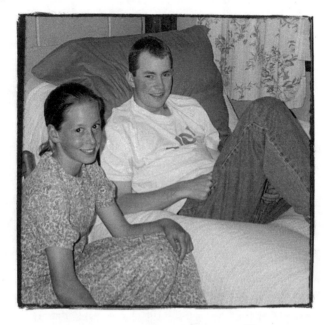

With Cynthia's sister Rhona

I can't just give up. I'm gonna do all I can to get through this." But now he said he realized that we weren't giving up. We were just deciding, finally, to listen to our hearts, be brave, and trust God. And *that's* when we found total peace – a peace that lasted throughout the remainder of our time together. Now we could put all our remaining energy into loving each other and everyone else in the community. We could use every minute we had left for that, and not worry about what might happen to us. I'll never forget how free I felt – like I could have almost flown. It was exciting, in a way, even though it was still hard.

Randy and Linda went to see Matt and Cynthia in the early afternoon and sensed the change immediately. "There was such a feeling of peace around them," Randy recalls.

Nevertheless, it was a difficult moment: "When they told us what they had decided, it was a relief, but it was also a shock. I guess the finality of it hit me: no more treatment for my son. He is going to die." "In a way," Randy confesses, "I was almost hoping that they would decide the opposite."

Musing on their flip-flopping emotions, Linda says: "We wanted to let go, but here we were once again, struggling against holding onto him. It's scary to think of making a mistake. You don't want to condemn your child. You start thinking, 'What if a new protocol would have worked?' But our overriding feeling *was* one of peace. It was as if Matt no longer belonged to us, but to God." Randy agrees: "We had turned a corner. Now we could concentrate on making him comfortable, and help make his last days or weeks as fulfilled as possible."

Gladys, Cynthia's mother, also sensed that an important line had been crossed, and remembers the firmness with which her daughter emerged from the morning's struggles: "Cynthia said to me, 'Mom, we are *not* going to have a lot of crying and weeping. We are going to make use of however many days we have left. What's important is that we love each other more, not that we live another fifty or sixty years.'"

And there wasn't a lot of crying. In fact, Jonathan notes that after Matt's decision to relinquish further chemo, he was almost radiant – "inwardly peaceful, and grateful for anything anyone did for him. He even seemed to be sleeping better." Moreover, though Matt still suffered greatly toward the end, the excruciating pain that had accompanied his cancer the first time around, in November, never returned.

7

BEFORE MORNING

IT WAS EARLY JUNE, and Matt was becoming frailer and more listless every day. For the fourth week in a row, his hacking cough got worse; he was shockingly thin; and abdominal distension was beginning to make breathing difficult. Though repeatedly offered supplemental oxygen, he mostly declined, saying he found it more bothersome than helpful. Thankfully, Matt was "cheerful, not at all depressed" as Jonathan noted. So was Cynthia. As she wrote to Christoph and his wife:

> Although it is continually hard, we are at peace, knowing that God must need Matt for a purpose and that I must stay down here and work for the same purpose. It is a very special time for us. I can't

explain how I feel…but sometimes it seems as if I get glimpses of where Matt might be going. When I look at him I don't see his body so much as his soul, and that is a very special thing to me.

All the same, it was still heartbreaking for her to watch her husband's health deteriorate. As Christoph put it, Matt's days were numbered, and every hour was precious. "Look into each other's eyes; laugh and cry," he advised her. "Most of all, pray that the God-given bond of love between you is strengthened and not weakened." Cynthia hung onto every word. She had felt that way since Matt's re-diagnosis on May 26, but now time was running out, and she was determined to make each moment count. In her own words:

Matt and I stayed together every minute of the day and talked about everything that we felt was important. I don't know how many times we would just lie on the bed and talk and wonder and imagine what Matt would be seeing and doing in a few days. Those were the most special moments we ever shared. Tears would stream down our faces, the excitement in us was so strong. It was just hard to think that we would not be allowed to go together – you have no idea how much I wanted to go – and that affected Matt keenly. He would look so excited and then he would look over at me and be totally torn apart, because he didn't want to leave me behind. He knew that he would have to, but he would tell me many times a day, "Cynthia, I can't believe I'm going to have to leave you."

Nights were the worst, so Cynthia often stayed up with Matt. One evening, though, she was so exhausted that she reluctantly asked Randy to stay with him: "It was around midnight, and I *had* to sleep, and Matt had always told me to get enough rest so that we could be together during the day," she says.

The next afternoon we were out on his golf cart, and out of the blue he said, "I'm sorry I got mad at you." I asked him what he was talking about. He said that after I had left our bedroom the night before, he had been angry, because he thought I couldn't handle seeing him sick. He said that if the days ahead were going to be anything like last November, then the real pain and suffering hadn't even started yet. He said, "How will you be able to stay with me then?"

He wasn't really mad at me, I think, just upset that I would have to see him suffer. I understood completely and told him I would always stay with him, no matter how bad it got. He was quiet for a moment, then looked at me and said, "Yeah, but they all said that in the hospital, too, and then they couldn't take it." Then he cried and told me how much he would need me. He said, "Just to be able to see your face will get me through it all."

Matt found relief from his deepest fears through praying, too, and Cynthia says the following prayer in particular (from a book he was reading by Søren Kierkegaard) gave him strength and comfort in his last days. Perhaps its honest acknowledgment of fear reassured him; perhaps its confident tone steadied him when everything began to swim before his eyes. Whatever it was, he read and re-read it – no, prayed it – with all his heart:

> We do not know the time and the place. Perhaps a long road still lies before us. But when strength is taken away from us; when exhaustion fogs our eyes so that we peer out as into a dark night, and restless desires stir within us, wild impatient longings, and the heart groans in fearful anticipation of what is coming – O God, fix in our hearts the conviction that also while we are living, we belong to you.

Armed with this certainty, he was able to look beyond his own suffering, and ultimately he agonized more over others than over himself. As Cynthia's father, Richard, recalls, "I was watching him one night toward the end, and he woke, hacking and heaving, but thinking of his wife. He said, "God, this cough is going to kill me…Whatever happens, be sure you look after Cynthia."

By the beginning of June, Matt was so frail that he was barely able to go out in his golf cart, though he still insisted on it. "It's my only means of escape," he told a friend. Remembering the painful last ride to a picnic spot about half a mile from their house, Linda says, "A few days before he died he drove us out to the pond, and he was *so* careful. It felt like going in slow motion, and it just broke my heart. Earlier, he used to drive fast. He'd even race Ruth, an elderly neighbor of ours who uses a motorized scooter. Now he doesn't even pass anyone…"

A day or so later, Matt asked his father what dying would be like. As Randy remembers their conversation:

> We were sitting there alone, and he asked me if I knew how it would be in the end. All I could tell him was that we would be with him, and Jesus would be too. We talked about being ready to face God. Matt was crying, and my heart was breaking. Then I looked deep into his eyes, and there was a profound understanding between us. We both knew what would happen. We knew that nothing would be able to separate him or me from the love of God. It was such a deep experience, yet behind our tears there was also the unspoken pain that we would still have to face a separation in this world.

If the thought of watching Matt suffer had been Cynthia's greatest fear thus far, it was now this one – being separated – that began to loom largest. Yes, she'd be there for him until his dying breath. But after that, he'd no longer be there for *her* – just when she'd need him more than ever before. Contemplating the day they'd no longer be together, she asked Matt to write down something she could hold onto after he was gone:

I don't think Matt would have done it on his own. It wasn't his kind of thing. He kept putting it off, and I didn't like to remind him, because when I did, it would make us cry. So I didn't bring it up anymore. I figured that if he wanted to write, he would. Then, on his last afternoon, about twelve hours before he died, I was sitting with him and he started to cry. I asked him what the matter was.

He said, "I haven't written anything yet."

I said, "You don't have to do it today. You can do it tomorrow." He was really tired. I told him, "I want you to rest; there's no way you can manage it today."

He said, "Well, I'll be too tired tomorrow."

I tried to talk him out of it. I said, "I don't want you to do it. It will be too hard, and if you cry you won't be able to breathe. I know what you feel inside. You don't have to write anything." But he insisted. He even wanted to type it first, and then make me a clean copy by hand. I said, "That's too much work. Just do something short, and write it once. It doesn't matter if you have to cross out and erase."

After Cynthia left the room, Matt wrote her a letter. It took him the next two hours, and even then he didn't really finish. "He didn't sign it or write 'Love, Matt' or anything," Cynthia says. "But he did it," she adds defiantly. Excerpts follow:

June 8, 2000

My dearest Cynthia,

I suppose you could call this The Never-Ending Story, because as far as we are both concerned, I think our lives will remain intertwined…

You know, we had so much fun together in the short time we were married, I almost have started to believe Christoph – that it isn't how long you are married, but what you do with your time. And I can assure you I feel that we have done just about all we can to make this bond between us the best it could be…

When I am gone, you will have to continue on with your life, just as I am sure that you would want me to if you were in my shoes. I certainly won't give you any suggestions, because you can figure things out for yourself…

One thing I want to impress on you: I hope you never become bitter at God or question why things turned out the way they did. None of us can understand why God does what he does, and in the end, perhaps more was done for his kingdom than we will ever be able to imagine. So you must promise me that, no matter what happens…

You know, this is very difficult for me to write, I guess mainly because it means I am saying farewell to you in a way I couldn't say it face to face. The fact is, though, I am excited to go to Jesus and also to see you there when it is your time, next year or in fifty. Who knows?

Always know that I will be watching out for you wherever or whatever you are doing. At least that is how I am hoping it works. And of course I can never thank you enough for being there for me (I tried to do the same for you). Without you I don't think I would have made it this far…

Well, I don't know what else to write right now, although I may add some more later. Most of all know that you are first and foremost in the love of God and the church and that I am just one step behind you all the time…

Later the same evening, Matt asked to be taken outdoors. A reunion of several hundred youth – many of them friends and former classmates from out of state – had been scheduled for the weekend, and now they were gathering around a bonfire. He was eager to meet as many as he could. Randy remembers:

Matt insisted on going out, though we weren't sure he would make it. He was finding it harder and harder to breathe, and he'd been using oxygen a whole day already. But since we had a portable tank, we decided to let him go, even if he only lasted a few minutes.

He didn't have a wheelchair – he'd refused one up till then – but we borrowed one from a neighbor and got him into it, and I pushed him outdoors, with Cynthia's dad carrying the oxygen tank.

The crowd took forever to assemble. "Hey, how are you?" "Where are you living these days?" "What've you been up to?" The buzz went on and on as people mingled on the grass. Then Matt was wheeled into the circle, and suddenly everyone fell silent. The change in atmosphere was immediate. "It was as if all our hearts went out to Matt at once," says a friend. "No one said it, but we all knew that he had come out especially to say goodbye. We just sat there, drinking it in, and those of us near him tried to keep from crying."

Then someone started a song, and everyone joined in. Randy glanced over at Matt. Moments earlier he had been gasping for breath; now he was quiet. "His face was more peaceful than I had ever seen it," Randy remembers. "He was alert; his eyes were bright; he gazed intently at this person and then that one – it was as if he was taking in each one for the last time."

Someone started a second song, and then a third, and Matt began to clap along with the singing. Cynthia was taken by surprise: "He had so little energy," she says, "and it was so unlike him to clap. And he was way off beat. But when I looked at his face he was happy, smiling like a little boy, totally unselfconscious. That's when I thought: he is ready to go."

Cynthia was not the only one to see Matt in this way. In fact, during the weeks that followed his death, many in the community made the same observation. They were also reminded of Jesus' words, "Unless you become like a little child, you cannot enter the kingdom of heaven."

Matt's cancer had ravaged his body terribly over the past half year. But what of his spirit? If anything, it had renewed him and brought the long-lost child in him back to the surface. At the outset, he had been stripped of his arrogance and invincibility, and brought to his knees – to confession and a clear conscience. Now he was coming full circle, regaining his childlike innocence and accepting for the first time his utter dependence on others.

Recalling Matt's last evening, an old classmate says:

After a few more songs, someone said that we probably ought to let Matt get home. Matt didn't want to, though. He stayed for almost two more hours, sitting there in his wheelchair, and shaking hands all around. He even managed a few words here and there. I think he'd been storing up all day for it.

At one point Randy and Linda were reminiscing about old times, when Matt and the rest of us were in grade school. "Remember when…?" Chuckle. It was wrenching. We were torn between our love of Matt and our fear that he was dying, and we didn't know what to do or say. Matt seemed to understand, though, and that helped. Once or twice his parents tried to convince him to leave, but he mumbled through his oxygen mask, "There's no more time to rest." Finally they got him to head back indoors.

Back in the apartment, Randy helped Matt shower, after which he ate a little yogurt. Jonathan, who had dropped in, gave him something to help him sleep better:

> Despite his medication Matt was breathing sixty to eighty times a minute, as he had been for the last day or so. I wondered how long he could keep going like that. He was physically fit, and I worried that he might still have a long road ahead of him. At the same time, I knew he could go at any moment. We had to be ready for either.

As Jonathan left, he wished Matt a peaceful night. Matt looked him straight in the eye and replied, "I wish *you* a peaceful night." In Randy's words:

> After that, about 9:30, we got him to bed. We agreed that Cynthia should rest, and that I would spend the

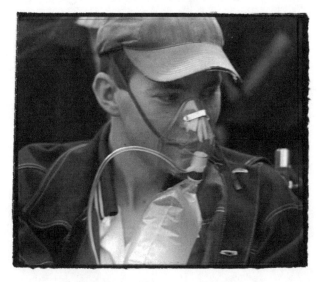

Saying good-bye

first half of the night with Matt. Linda would do the second half. For the first few hours I sat beside him, my hand on his arm, as he drifted in and out of sleep. He was peaceful, though on oxygen.

Then, around 11:30, he became restless and quite anxious, pulling at his oxygen mask and fighting for air. Cynthia got up, and Linda came in to be with us, too, and we gave him another dose of morphine. We also said a prayer for him.

Shortly after midnight Matt became very thirsty and took a few sips of water. He kept adjusting the oxygen mask and trying to talk. After a few minutes of struggling with the mask, he took it off and set it on the edge of the bed. Cynthia remembers:

> It was awful watching him, though we assured him that we were right there. A few weeks earlier he had told me, "Cynthia, I can take any amount of pain, but not being able to breathe…it's like I'm drowning. I keep getting pushed under."
>
> Then one day I came into our bedroom and found him reading the Psalms and crying, and he said that what scared him the most was thinking about when they would take his oxygen mask off. I asked him what he meant. He told me he was worried that eventually things would get so bad that we would just decide to take off his mask and let him

go. I reassured him we wouldn't do that. But I don't think I had any idea how bad it would get.

Anyway, now his mask was off, and I felt our prayers had been answered. Nobody had removed it. He had taken it off himself.

Nick, Matt's younger brother, will never forget that moment:

It was scary for me when Matt took off his mask, because he was frantic for breath and I felt like he was throwing away his last chance. I guess I was expecting him to die all of a sudden. But I don't think it was scary for him. Maybe for a moment or two before he took it off, when he was thinking about it. Maybe. But once he took it off, he didn't reach for it again. It was like a decision that he made – like he was saying, "I can do it on my own." It was an amazing thing.

By 1:00 Matt was more peaceful. To quote Jonathan's journal:

Cynthia asked for me to come downstairs again. When I got there Matt's breathing was still very rapid and shallow, but there was a palpable peace in the room. Seeing the tremendous effort of his breathing, even more than an hour or two previously, my first impulse was to pray that his soul be released from his body. But then I saw the look of acceptance on his face, and the peace – actually a radiant joy – on the faces of Cynthia and his parents, and I had to realize once again that God knows the hour of each one of us, and we have to be patient for it.

It was around then that we began to sing to him: songs of redemption and of heaven – childlike songs. We spent much of the next hour in silence, though at one point Randy prayed. We also spoke short words of encouragement to him. Matt asked for water now and then, and several times he gave us one of his asymmetrical little smiles. He also thanked us for singing to him: "It's not such a big deal, but it's the best thing right now for me."

Although intermittently confused, he showed touches of humor and made several lucid comments between labored breaths. At one point he groaned, "Doctors" (as Nick commented, that was so *him*), and then mumbled, "Where is Jonathan?" Later he said something about "going" somewhere, and I replied, "Yes, you can go, Jesus will take you!"

"But it's so hard!" he responded.

I said, "Don't cling to us. Cling to God!"

"I'm trying," he said, "but I don't know what to do next. It's so unfamiliar!"

To that, Cynthia said, "Yes, but you are going before us, and then you can tell us how to get there!"

Randy added that he should pray for us and fight for us from the other side.

Shortly afterward he said, "We must think of others in my situation who don't have support." He then asked, "Is there no book in the house?" Randy and Richard then read him several passages from the New Testament – words of encouragement and hope and peace. But Matt called out, "What Dad wrote!" meaning several other passages that Randy had highlighted for him a few days before. "If you don't understand it, you can always ask Charles!" he added, referring to a friend with a seminary degree.

Randy then read most of Romans, chapter 8, aloud. Just as he was finishing, Matt said, "Maybe Jesus will come!" Several of us responded, "He *will* come!"

Later Cynthia told him she was slipping out of the room for a moment, and he said quite loudly, "Can't wait much longer!"

Around 3 o'clock Jacob and his wife came in. Over the next half hour, Matt's breathing became more labored, though every few minutes he would say something. Sometimes it was just one word; sometimes a whole sentence, but hurriedly spoken between gasps, and hard to understand. His eyes were open, but he didn't seem to see us any more: "This is a great struggle…You don't know how tired

I am! Pathetic…Don't focus on…but on the spiritual." This last, I'm sure, was a reference to what he had said so many times over the last two weeks: "We have to focus on God, not the disease."

Later he said, among other things, "Gotta go… Jesus…Amazing! Very real…" Then, after quite a pause, he said, "I feel real bad, but I can't do anything about it now." Jacob assured him that whatever it was, he was forgiven; that God would take him; and that it would be very soon. Matt then asked for water, and said, "Gonna go very shortly…One of my best days…"

Around 3:30 he developed an intonation at every breath, and after that he didn't speak anymore. Neither did we. It was terribly hard to see and hear him breathing like that, and many silent prayers went up as intercession for his soul.

At 4:15 his breathing grew slower, though not irregular, and his color more pallid. We could hold back our tears no longer. His breathing became even calmer and quieter. We all sensed it, and drew together, with hands on each other's shoulders. Cynthia was at his head, Linda and Nick were at his side, and Randy sat on the end of his bed, holding one of his hands and stroking his leg.

Then, at 4:30, the end came. It was mercifully peaceful. Cynthia had one hand in Matt's, and the other over his heart, and as she slowly felt his life slip away, the rest of us drew in around her. At the final moment, Gladys put her arms around her daughter, and Linda reached out to hold Randy. Matt let out two great shuddering breaths. Linda and Cynthia called out to him. Then he was gone.

Cynthia, choking with sobs, put her face to Matt's cheek. Suddenly she looked up. "Dad, Mom, I hear singing." There was a moment of quiet. "Don't you hear it?" she asked. "No," said Gladys. Cynthia tilted her head to one side, puzzled: "Someone is singing outside." (Afterwards Cynthia told her parents, "I'm not mental or anything, but I heard this tremendous music. It was like singing, but it wasn't. It was a loud, rushing noise. Like I had gone halfway there with Matt.")

Now it was nearing 5:00 a.m., and the family was dressing the body. Afterwards Matt looked his familiar self, lying on a white sheet in his favorite clothes – blue jeans, a checkered flannel shirt, and a faded purple cap. His black denim jacket, made by Cynthia, lay at his head.

Jonathan left the house. Stepping into the dewy cold, he took in the first signs of light in the East, and the deafening, twittering chorus of birds. The dawn was just beginning.

8

TIES THAT BIND

THE AFTERNOON after Matt died, a festival was held on the lawn outside his room. It was a perfect summer day, and there were balloons and pony rides, food booths and guessing games, races, and a waterslide. And hundreds of boys and girls.

Planned for weeks in advance, the Children's Fest is an annual event at every Bruderhof, and in that way, this one was no different. Given its timing, however, it will always stand out for those who were there. After all, the busiest corner of the temporary fair grounds was not the ice cream stand, but the entrance to Matt's apartment where, on a table next to it, the white lid of his casket slowly filled with handwritten messages of farewell.

All afternoon the crowd wound their way inside the house and down the hall to Matt – most of them silent, some in tears, and several pulled by four, five, and six-year-olds eager to say goodbye to the lanky kid who used to toss a frisbee with them or catch their runaway balls. But it wasn't a line of mourners by any means, not if you judged it by the strange radiance on the faces of many as they came back out of the house. And even though a few children came in licking cones, no one – including Cynthia – seemed the slightest bit uncomfortable.

Far from being incongruous with the rest of the weekend, the festival was a better tribute than anything one could have planned for Matt. An affirmation of life, it honored his struggle against death; a celebration, it reminded everyone that his terrible suffering was over, and that he was finally at rest. As Mina, a friend who went to college with Matt and later worked in the same office with him, put it, "To people who weren't there it might seem strange, but Matt's death did *not* create a feeling of heaviness or sadness, at least not for those of us who were around him for the duration of his illness. He had fought for six whole months, and now the battle was over. There were tears, of course, but no one I know was depressed. If anything, many of us felt a sense of tremendous release – even joy."

All in all, the event was a powerful reminder of the way life's many threads are tied into one whole, even though they often seem to run in different or even opposing directions. Laughter and tears, misery and joy, the agony of separation and the deep bonds that shared suffering can bring – they were all one.

In fact, the spirit of oneness that Matt's death drew forth was noticeable throughout his illness. Matt and Cynthia did not suffer together in a vacuum, but in the context of an entire community who suffered with them and on their behalf. And because their pain was shared by others, it was somehow robbed of its power to end in despair.

Around Christmas, when Matt's hair began to fall out, dozens of young men in the community had shaved their heads as a sign of solidarity, and here and there even a child begged to have his hair cut too. On a deeper level, the shock of seeing a healthy young man laid low by an incurable disease gave many pause about the meaning of life – and the positive sides of vulnerability and interdependence. And it didn't stop with Matt's death. As Jonathan noted a week or so later:

> I am overwhelmed by the closeness, the unity, the togetherness among brothers and sisters in these days. The fact that physical healing was not given to Matt has driven us all to prayer and to God so much

more than we might have been. We have talked, laughed, prayed, and wept together and found each other in ways that I didn't know was possible. I still grieve for Matt. There are still times when I cry – I don't even know why. But the victory of his last night remains.

Those who were with Matt when he died point out that the peace he experienced in his final hours was not something that just fell into his lap. In Jonathan's words, "It was fought for at great cost to himself over months and years, though especially during his last week."

This fight took shape in very concrete ways. As Randy and Linda put it, Matt was no saint. Nor did he see eye to eye with them on everything, especially when, as a twenty-two-year-old, he felt that they were overly concerned about his inner well-being. Three days before he died, for instance, someone brought a handful of rental movies for him to watch, and when his parents voiced their worry that he might fritter away his last hours on earth entertaining himself, they found themselves embroiled in a classic family fight. As Linda remembers it:

People brought videos for Matt to watch throughout his illness, and though I knew they meant well, I was always a little uncomfortable with it. It wasn't a question of the movies – though some of the stuff

he watched wasn't all that great. I just felt he was using them too often, as an easy out, a means of escape
from reality. I didn't think it was healthy.

To be honest, I felt the same about a lot of
other things people gave him, especially after he
was diagnosed the first time. There was beer, hard
liquor, CD's – dozens of them – posters, headphones, cordless headphones, a radio, a new stereo
system with six speakers, a Rio player for down-
loading music from the Internet, and on and on.

I remember talking about it with Randy, and
wondering: Is this really the best way of showing
kindness to someone with cancer? Dumping a lot of
junk on him? Sure, we knew it would comfort him in
a material way. But ultimately, these gifts were just
things – things to divert him from real life-and-death
issues he needed to face. Matt felt the same way about
most of it, and at one point he cleared a lot of that
stuff out of his room.

Anyway, Randy and I were concerned that Matt
would want to spend what turned out to be one of
the last afternoons of his life watching movies. But
he did not agree with us at all. He said, "I just want
to be able to laugh and forget about things for a few
hours! How can you be my moral compass now?" He
was so mad.

I was in tears, because I was thinking, "Here's
this poor kid who just wants to escape for a few

hours. Doesn't he have a right to do that – to have a little fun?" Besides, I had just read this book on death and dying where the author talks about how important it is to create peace around a dying person. The book said, "no family quarrels," and here we were arguing. It just tore me apart.

I love to watch movies myself. But I also felt, and still feel, that it's too easy to escape (or let your children escape) so you don't have to deal with things that are hard. I'm not just talking about cancer. Whenever you are in a struggle – any struggle – you need to set your sights on the things that will strengthen you, not distract you, if you're going to make it through.

On the other hand, I thought, "Matt's upset because I am being too moralistic. I have to listen to him. Maybe he's saying something I really need to take to heart…After all, he's dying! But he's still my son, and I know that escaping is not good for him. Can I risk *not* saying something that might be vitally important for him?" It was one of the hardest moments I have ever faced.

From Cynthia's perspective, the conflict was just as hard:

I knew they had a good point, and Matt did too. Later, in our room, he said, "They're always right, but I don't think they understand." I was fuming. I said, "Look at all the stuff that's happened to us; and we're still so young. No one else knows what it's like." But after a while we calmed down. Matt said that deep down he knew that watching movies was a waste of time when he had so little time left, and that he actually wanted to spend it with other people, and then he went and told his parents he understood. He even thanked them for not giving in.

If the "video thing," as Randy calls it, makes Matt's relations with his parents sound like they were strained, friends say nothing could be further from the truth. If anything, the family's honesty in dealing with differences seems to have held them together through the roughest spots of Matt's last six months and made them love each other more deeply than ever. Further, as Linda points out, fighting "for Matt's soul" was the only kind of fighting she could do for him, because much as she wanted to, she couldn't do anything about his cancer. Most of all, though, she simply loved him – with everything she had:

> When Matt and Nick were little, about six months old, they would get viral infections and high fevers that would last four or five days, and when your children are sick like that, you hold them a lot. I also hummed and sang to them a lot. It didn't matter what I would sing – whatever it was, there was so much love in it, it just flowed from Mom to child as I held them. I spent so many hours just rocking

one or the other in my arms, doing that. Sometimes, that's about all you can do, and sometimes it's just as good, or better, than medicine.

A few days before Matt died, I was sitting by his bedside alone with him, just holding his hand, and he had his eyes shut. He was so tired, and I started to hum this evening song – "Good night to you all, and sweet be your sleep…" I got about halfway through when the tears just started streaming down Matt's face, even though his eyes were shut. I started crying too, and we just held each other tight. I stroked his head and cheek, and told him that we would be with him all the time, that we would be with him until he left us, and that we loved him so much.

I sang to Matt one other time when he was sick, and that was the night he died. I was sitting next to him, holding his hand, and I just started to hum to him. There were other people in the room, but it felt like long ago – like it was just the two of us there. Just mother and child. I thought of "Billy Boy," which had been one of his and Nick's favorites when they were little. It was the standard "sick" song in our house, one I always sang to comfort them and make them feel better.

Then I remembered that I wasn't alone with Matt, so I chose a different song and started humming. I can't say if it made Matt feel better, but it made me feel that I was doing all I could for him, even if it was such a little thing. Later, Matt asked if we could sing. We did – song after song – but I felt *so* bad that he had had to ask. Why hadn't I thought of it?

Now that Matt's gone I just cry and cry when I hear those songs we sang to him on his last night. I can't sing them anymore. I don't know if I will ever be able to sing them again.

Linda says that even a mundane act like cutting her son's hair gained new meaning for her toward the end of his life, because it left her wondering how many more times she'd still be able to do it for him:

I cut Matt's hair twice while he was sick; I'd done it ever since he was two years old. The first time was after the chemo started to make his hair fall out. He asked me to trim it so that he could shave it close afterward. I started, but after a few strokes with the electric hair cutter, I had to quit. I was in tears. There was the scar on the back of his head, the one he got when he was two from falling backward on cement steps. My little one – so big – but still my little one – I was shaving his head because he had cancer, and the chemo was making it all fall out. I told Randy that I couldn't do it. He had to take over.

The second time was about a week before he died. He said his hair was getting too long around the ears. He never liked that, and even if I didn't think it needed cutting, he always ended up convinc-

ing me to do it. It tugged at my heart. This would be
the last time. Stop – don't think – just do it. Matt
was so tired; I knew he'd need to lie down again
soon. His hair was so soft after growing back from
the chemo. It hadn't been that soft since he was little.
I had to resist the urge to stroke it: "He's big; he's an
adult; he's married," I told myself. But he was still my
little one deep down – and always will be…

All he needs is a trim. Should be simple and fast.
But he's weak, weaving and nodding a bit. I want to
make it fast. Now everything's done but the back. I
use the electric cutter with the right guard and – Oh,
there are big bumps on the back of his head! The
nodes are so swollen. I almost can't finish. My poor
honey! He must know they are there, and he must
know that I know. I feel them with my fingers…

The simple act of sitting together in silence, too,
gained new significance for Randy and Linda during
Matt's illness, and after his death it was a vital part of
their healing as they began to grieve. "A caring silence
can enter deeper into our memory than many caring
words," author Henri Nouwen writes in a book Linda
read during Matt's illness, and for her, at least, it has
proved true.

Just the previous summer, Randy and Linda had
spent several days visiting Brad and Misty Bernall,
whose daughter Cassie was one of thirteen students

killed in the infamous Columbine High School massacre of April 20, 1999. Speaking of the time she spent
with Misty, Linda remembers weeding the family gar-
den with her, and trying to comfort her, though ad-
mitting that there was no way she could understand
what Misty was going through. "There was a lot of
silence between us," Linda recalls. "At times I understood the need for it; other times I worried that she
was upset with me."

Now Linda has a deeper appreciation for Misty's
inability to chatter. "Because there just aren't any
words that will make you feel better, silence is often
what you want and need most. It heals." She goes on:

> I knew Misty was thinking of me over the last six
> months we had with Matt, and I knew she was hurt-
> ing – for herself again, and for me. There were no
> words between us, but I felt close to her in our si-
> lence. A few times I picked up the phone to call her
> but just couldn't. There weren't any words to say. If I
> could have seen her, there would have been tears, but
> I don't think there would have been any words.
>
> Three weeks after Matt died, Brad and Misty
> sent us a beautiful flower arrangement, with a card
> saying "We're praying for you." I thought of how
> hard it must have been for her to call the florist, and
> on the spur of the moment, I decided to call and
> thank her. I thought I'd be okay on the phone this
> time.

I called and got her voice mail, so I said, "Hi, Misty, this is Linda. Thanks for the flowers. I love you." Then I broke down. Her pain – my pain – what was there to say? I choked and quickly hung up.

The day before Matt died, Linda spent a long time in her living room, sitting quietly on the couch with a friend. A few days later, the same friend came back with another woman, and the three of them held hands as the tears trickled down their checks. "There is nothing more special than being with someone in total silence, and knowing that you feel each other's hurt," says Linda. "It is an expression of deep love."

The day after the funeral, Randy experienced the same when he and Jonathan packed up medical equipment, returned medications, and closed Matt's charts. As Randy stepped into Jonathan's exam room with the last box, he found him weeping, gave him a hug, and slipped out again. Later, at home, Linda, who was helping Cynthia to tidy their apartment, asked Randy to clean out a drawer. Opening it, he found Matt's shaving things, and it was his turn to break down and cry. Still, Randy says there were plenty of things to laugh over too. "You've got to do both – laugh and cry. It's all part of the same picture."

Illness often drives couples apart, and even with a supportive community around them, Randy and Linda found their marriage subjected to difficult tests.

Ultimately, however, Matt's cancer drew them together. Looking back on the nerve-wracking weeks they spent in Australia between his final round of chemo in March and his re-diagnosis in May, Linda says:

> The strain was immense. On one hand, I wanted to be back home in Pennsylvania with Matt; on the other, he was now a married man, and I knew I shouldn't cling to him. Sometimes I just fell apart. And then, when I tried to talk to Randy about it, I just never got the response I wanted. Who knows what response I wanted anyway? Maybe I was too emotional. Maybe he was not emotional enough. Neither of us was right or wrong. But we weren't connecting, so we couldn't help each other or comfort each other.
>
> Then, about two weeks before we flew back home, it all changed. I don't know how it happened, but somehow, through Matt and Cynthia's suffering, through our suffering, God came to us and helped us. I could talk to Randy, and he could listen. I could cry, and he could hold me and cry too. I have never felt such a love between us – and it has stayed with us. If God had not given us this unity of heart in Australia, and we had returned to be with Matt in his final days without it, I don't know how we would have coped. It still makes me cry today, because this love is something that we have wanted in our mar-

riage from day one, and it has finally been given to us. But to find it, we had to lose Matt.

From Randy's perspective:

I kept my concerns about Matt's situation bottled up because I was concerned that Linda was not handling things. The fact that I didn't allow her to fully share her worries with me created a lot of tension. She needed someone to confide in, someone who could identify with her fears. She needed me.

Then came that breakthrough, when I finally stopped keeping a wall up between us; when I allowed myself to become vulnerable. I realized that drawing into a shell in the face of Matt's illness could rip our marriage apart. We both knew of marriages where the pain and struggle that should draw husband and wife closer together actually did the opposite. Couples were driven apart by holding their feelings inside, distancing themselves from one another, and speculating about what the other one thought or felt.

A big part of the challenge was simply dealing with our emotions: one day we could look at a photo of Matt and smile. The next day we'd see the same one and totally fall apart. But to admit to yourself that you are just a plain, ordinary, weak person, and that you aren't coping, and that it's okay – that is a

tremendous relief. After you do that, you no longer
feel the need to deny or suppress your emotions, or
to worry if they are abnormal or wrong. If you need
to cry, cry.

Anyway, once we were able to do this, and to see
our stress mirrored in each other, we could share it
openly together. We held each other and wept for as
long as we needed to. And then we could say, "Well,
that's enough for now, let's go on."

Commenting on the way Matt's illness brought
his parents closer to each other, Nick says it also
strengthened his own interaction with them – and
others:

Before, it was hard to talk about a lot of things. Now
I feel the need to be totally honest, to say what I feel
instead of keeping it inside. I mean, who knows who
could die next? Besides, our little outward shells
don't protect us, they just separate us. They don't
need to be there.

Grieving is hard, but it can bring you together
with other people. My dad and I helped dress Matt
after he died, and Jonathan made us feel that we
could help, although he said we didn't have to if
we'd rather not. It was good to be incorporated
into things instead of stepping back and watching
everything happen. I think you end up feeling
numb when you're just an observer.

It was scary to put on Matt's clothes and to feel his limp body, but at the same time I wouldn't have missed it – it was like a last service of love for him. If you just walk away from something, there's not much more you can say than, "Wow, what just happened?" But if you can say, "I did something, and I *know* what I just did," it has meaning.

Actually, the whole last week I spent with Matt was so meaningful. And I know it sounds weird to say it, but it was worth a lifetime. Really. That's not just a cliché. And his last night was definitely the best time I've ever spent with him, especially the last twenty minutes. It was hard. But it was also good. *All* good. I could smile the whole way through, even while crying. I felt like there was this good energy.

Moreover, Nick says that his brother's death left him with a new appreciation for the reality of an invisible world beyond time and space:

Right after Matt went, Cynthia said that she was hearing music or something. And it's funny, but I swear that when she said that, I listened and I could hear something too. It's weird, but it's brought me to a different level of thinking about everything. I think we're so much more interconnected with the other world, as you might call it, than we sometimes assume. We have our little plans and go on with our little lives, but there's always that connection.

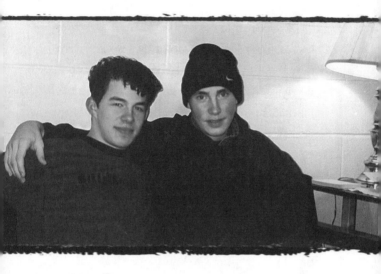

Brothers forever

It's a connection that's given Cynthia plenty to think about, though she's hesitant to speak about it casually. She will say this, however: if Matt's illness enlarged her vision of reality or deepened her faith, it happened only because he allowed himself to be chiseled and transformed by his suffering – and challenged her to do the same:

> We had both been kind of loud, superficial people before Matt got cancer. And though Matt stayed who he was in many ways, he knew – especially after he got sick the second time – that there just wasn't time for all that. Instead, he took time to be there for other people. He'd spend time with kids, and sit them on his lap.
>
> There was a sort of spiritual leadership, too, that I hadn't seen in him before, and a firmness. He didn't talk anymore about things that didn't matter. Everything he said had a purpose, and he said it with conviction, even excitement. His prayers, the little things we read aloud together – every word was meaningful. There was no time to be inwardly asleep.
>
> Sometimes the other world was very close and tangible. We didn't have to talk about it – we could feel its power and peace, and that was all we needed to assure us that God knew best, and that everything would be all right in the end.

A couple of days before he died, we shared one of those silent moments when we were both trying to grasp the fact that we would soon be separated. Then I looked at him and told him how much it would encourage me to know that he was watching over me down here.

He said, "I hope that's how it works, because I would be sad if I couldn't see you."

I said I wished that he could be a little angel by my side – just mine.

He replied in a very determined voice, "I won't be your little angel. I'll be the biggest angel there is!"

Toward the end, the spiritual change in him became even more noticeable. It's hard to explain. But every time I looked at him I felt I was seeing more than I had seen before. It was like I was looking through him, and that I could catch a glimpse of where he was going. When our eyes met, we both knew and saw the same thing. He did not belong anymore to this world. It was as if he was already at home in a different place far, far away – as if he was already becoming my angel.

I once told him that he was changing. I couldn't tell him what I really meant; I just said I knew he was still Matt, and always would be, but that he was changing inside. He started to cry. He told me he wasn't sure he wanted to change. That is often how we both felt. It was such a special thing that was happening to us, yet we hadn't asked for it, and a part of us was still rebelling against it. I feel now that we were struggling to accept God's will. It's a fight I'm still waging to this day.

9

NEW SEEDS

NO MATTER the circumstances when someone dies, the same clichés get dusted off. Perhaps it is because we are afraid of hurting the bereaved by saying "the wrong thing." Perhaps we are too choked with emotion to even know what we really think. But there may be a deeper reason. Many of us, it seems, are so uncomfortable with the thought of death that we are happy to skirt the subject entirely by means of tried-and-true phrases. As one of Matt's friends put it after Matt died, we often treat the death of another person like a speed bump: "You slow down because you have to, but once you're over it, you pick up again right away."

It is simply a fact that in most parts of society today, death is viewed chiefly as an unfortunate disruption of the good life. It is a foolhardy view, not only because it will not shield us from anguish when death does strike – as it inevitably must – but also because it prevents us from finding the potential meaning that every loss carries. In Randy's words:

> It's a great temptation to throw oneself back into one's work, one's daily rhythm, or whatever – to "move on." But you *cannot* just move on if you want to take in the death of a person you love. Look at Matt: God spoke through his illness, and Linda and I don't want to "get over it." We want to be changed and challenged for the rest of our lives. Moving on as soon as we can might limit our pain, but will it bring full healing? We don't think so.

Jen, a close friend of Matt's brother, Nick, lost her brother, Jimmy, three years ago. Jimmy was sixteen and died of a drug overdose, and Jen was his only sibling. Yet when she took longer to grieve for him than others did, she was made to feel guilty:

> I tried to explain that I was not in denial, but I felt that people never really understood me. It seemed like they expected my life to be "normal" again. I often went through times of sadness, bitterness, and other painful emotions, but people were uncomfortable with this. I was so alone.
>
> Six months after Jimmy's death, a good friend of his died. I felt so much pain. But when I told one of

my friends how I was feeling, he said he was worried for me. He thought I should have been over "all of that" by now – which pressured me to feel the same.

I feel like I mourned my brother and his friend in isolation and confusion. I tried to gain meaning from their deaths, but it was very hard. Everyone just kept talking about how they shouldn't have died.

By upsetting our equanimity, every death reminds us that like it or not, life is not in our hands. It is a disquieting thought, especially when (as in Matt's case) we have managed to forestall dying for some time. But it is a vital one as well. In Linda's words:

Suffering cannot be put off forever, and when it comes, there is no way around the pain. Maybe that knowledge only comes with age and experience. But if I ever have to go through it again in my life, I hope I have grasped it. Life is *hard,* and there are some things that hurt – no matter how much you try to smooth them over or make them nicer. You might as well hit suffering head on when it comes your way, because it won't just disappear.

For Cynthia, this truth came into focus most sharply after Matt died, when her grief enveloped her in such a way that she had no choice but to deal with it. At first she seemed numbed by her pain, then beside herself with desperation. Finally, returning to the

cabin where she and Matt had spent their honey-
moon five months before, she confronted her heartache in the place it hurt most:

As soon as I arrived, I felt ripped apart inside. Every
room I looked into held memories. I could hear what
Matt had said to me; I could see the look on his face; I
could feel how he had held me. And I knew only one
thing: Matt was gone and would never come back. I
have never felt so alone and so totally forsaken by God
and everyone else in my life. I was angry. All I wanted
was for Matt to come back, to talk to me, to be with
me again. And I wasn't sure if anybody would ever
understand how much we loved each other. I wanted
to run far away and leave everything behind, to hide
my anger and sorrow. I wanted to listen to God, but I
didn't know how I could possibly hear him when I
was in so much pain.

I felt like a kid too young to understand what
had happened, and too confused to know how I was
ever supposed to keep on living. I must have cried
for hours.

Finally I walked away from the house and down
to a nearby stream. I couldn't go back in. I sat next to
the rushing water, watched the fish jumping, and got
quiet. I remembered the promise I had made to Matt:
that I would never become bitter or angry with God,
even though I didn't understand his ways. And

suddenly I knew why I was there. It was the hardest place to be, but also the place that would bring me the deepest healing.

Despite such agonized soul-searching – or perhaps as a result of it – Cynthia says she understands exactly how Matt must have felt when he said at their wedding that he wouldn't trade his life for anyone else's: "That is just what I also feel, deep down," she says. Randy and Linda say the same. Matt's cancer tried them – like nothing else they have ever been through. Yet far from leaving them defeated and broken, it tested their mettle in a way that ultimately strengthened them. And this was true from the start. In Randy's words:

> After Matt first got ill we began reading together every evening from a book of prayers. The words seemed as if they'd been written just for us, and we were struck by how shallow our prayer life had been up till then. It seemed like we'd followed a ritual instead of having real conversations with God. We'd been skating along in life. Everything had been going fine. Then suddenly Matt had cancer. We knew God must be trying to say something to us.

Brian, a former college classmate of Matt's, says he was similarly affected:

> I've always been someone who didn't take prayer too seriously. I was often so unfocused, I didn't even really

know what I was praying for. Matt's illness changed all that. From the day I heard he had cancer until the day he died, I prayed for him, and I have never prayed so intensely. It consumed me, I guess you could say. Even now that he's gone, he's kept me focused. I still pray every day that he didn't die in vain.

Like Brian, hundreds of others in the community felt that their inner lives were deepened over the last six months of Matt's life. To some, especially friends and former classmates, it was simply a matter of his cancer. After all, his flight from the basketball court to the oncology unit was impossible to ignore, especially because it happened in the space of a week. And even if most twenty-somethings can count on a long life ahead, the very word cancer has a way of throwing the safest assumptions into question.

To others it was the change in Matt's outlook on life that gave them pause. He remained himself – "a wise-ass to the end," says a former classmate – and though his cancer sobered him, it never made him pious or otherworldly. All the same, Matt's suffering was a crucible of sorts. And by yielding to its flames and letting them refine him, he offered to those around him an unspoken challenge to do the same.

Discussing this challenge at a member's meeting just a week before Matt died, his old high school mentor, Dave, proposed that it be acknowledged in some way. "Ever since Matt got sick," he said hesitat-

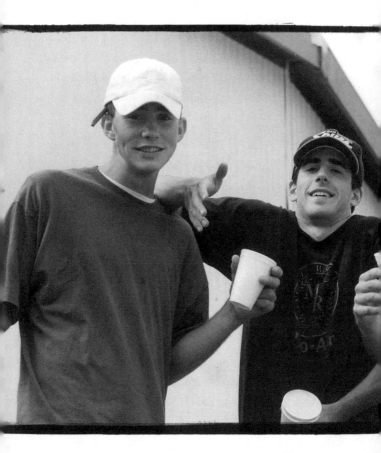

Hanging out with Brian

ingly, "I've felt that God wanted something else for him – something more than being a computer programmer. I think God wants to speak to us through him." Dave's words resonated with others, and by the end of the meeting, a unanimous decision had been made to ordain Matt a "servant" (as pastors of the Bruderhof are called) the same evening.

One person who was touched in a special way by Matt was a former college roommate, Reuben, who had since moved to California. When Reuben first heard that Matt had cancer, he was devastated. Later, however, feeling unable to deal with such bad news, he tried to brush it off. But he couldn't. How could he, when a friend had just received what amounted to a death sentence?

For the first time in years, Reuben found himself jolted out of his daily rhythm – and distraught enough over its emptiness to be driven to his knees. Within days he decided to take time off from his job and move to Pennsylvania in order to care for Matt; a week later he was flying out of L.A. As he later explained, "Matt's cancer made it clear to me that I needed to change, drastically. Through him God was trying to tell me to follow Him."

Eileen, too, went to school with Matt, and was living in Philadelphia when she heard about his cancer. The news came via an e-mail from Reuben, and on detecting its effect on him, she was wary. Determined not to get "emotional," as she later put it, she simultaneously sensed that God was stopping her in her tracks, and though she protested to a friend that "I'm *not* going to have a conversion over this," she did, anyway.

Visiting Matt around Christmas at the Bruderhof where they had both grown up (like Matt, she had moved there as a child), Eileen was bowled over by the transformation he had undergone. "This was not the Matt I'd gone to WVU with," she says. "He was quiet. He'd listen. He was positive and encouraging…I think he'd finally found a focus and given his life to God."

On the last day of May – almost two years after Matt himself had been baptized – Reuben and seven other young men and women took the same step. As Reuben explains:

> I'll never fully understand how Matt's life changed me – just that it did. Through his suffering, illness and death, I was changed in some way. That's why I decided to get baptized: I had to give my life to God. And through Matt I saw that that can't just be a theoretical thing. He knew that he was going to die shortly, and that brought home the reality of my own commitment.
>
> In the New Testament it says that you should lay down your life for your brother, and the way I look at it, Matt laid down his life for me. Without him I might have never found God.

Reuben asked Matt to perform the baptisms, and though he barely had strength to stand, he did – pouring water over each of the seven as a sign of cleansing, pronouncing to each one the forgiveness of their sins, and finally, blessing each with a prayer.

To anyone who was there, the torch-lit service, which was held outdoors at dusk, will be unforgettable. It is especially so for Maureen, who went through most of grade school and high school with Matt:

> If you had asked us back then which one in our class would have the greatest positive impact on other lives, no one would have picked Matt. Trust him to never be able to keep his mouth shut, to always have something sarcastic or flippant or risqué to say. He was a regular brat, a pain. At least that's how I knew him. But when God called him, he answered. No pedestal needed.

Darrell, a former roommate, agrees. Sitting, a few weeks after Matt's death, with a group of friends who were talking about how wonderful he was, Darrell jumped up, fuming: "Saint Matt this! Saint Matt that! I can't stand it." To him, the great thing about Matt was that he was "just a normal guy," and that God had used him anyway. To hold him up as a model or a hero would be to miss the whole point of his suffering, if not cheapen it.

The morning that Matt died, I went to see him. I just sort of stood by his bed and said to myself, "Well, Matt, you died for something. I'm going to make sure that I continue what you started." Matt's death was much more than just the death of a friend. It was something much greater than that. In a way, it left me confronted with a serious choice. Either I was going to serve God or I wasn't. It was that clear, and I had to make a choice *then*. I realized I couldn't run anymore. I couldn't hide anymore from God. My life just couldn't remain the same; things had to change.

Ironically, it seems that precisely in facing this same choice and deciding to live for God, Matt actually ceased to be a "normal guy," and began the long, arduous journey toward the remarkable night of his death. As Steve, Matt's pastor for the last ten years, explains it:

I know what people mean when they say Matt was no different from anyone else. He was far from perfect, and he never quite lost his wild side. But there's no question in my mind that once he submitted to God's will, he *did* deepen and change. Yes, there were times when he cried out in need and rebellion. But he had a clear conscience, and that gave him an incredible peace.

To me it's like this: Matt did not ask for it, but God put his finger on him.

Jesus says, "Unless a kernel of wheat falls to the ground and dies…it cannot send up new shoots." Matt did that – he surrendered his life to God. And look at the fruits!

Matt's death was actually a victory over death – over the powers of darkness, self-indulgence, and pride. It was a victory because it brought him and all of us around him back to the essentials; to the things of eternity – to the childlike spirit each of us needs in order to be part of the kingdom of God.

For Linda, losing Matt was unspeakably hard: "When you lose someone you're close to, especially if you're right there with him when he goes, the hurt and the shock are indescribably deep. I just don't know how we got through that time." Even so, she sees her son's death in the same light as Steve. It is the same for Cynthia: "I know there are going to be hard times ahead. But through Matt's death I have found a faith that no one can take away from me."

As for Randy, he says, "There is no way Matt's death was a defeat. It's true his cancer wasn't success-fully treated. But he found peace of heart, and in that sense he *was* healed – and so were many around him." And while Randy has lost a son, he says he has also lost something else: his fear of death. "Life still has its ups and downs. Some days you fall apart; other days you do okay. But being in that room with our son on the final night of his life has changed us forever. We finally saw that death need not be a frightening thing. It may be the last enemy, but it's not the end of the story."

CODA

ABOUT TWO WEEKS after Matt's death, Cynthia was sitting in an apartment at Woodcrest, the New York Bruderhof where she and her husband had first met. Thumbing through a book she had found on the shelf, a collection of essays by C. F. Blumhardt, she noticed that the margin of one page contained several arrows and the word "personal." The handwriting seemed familiar.

Turning to the front to see whose book it was, Cynthia started at the name on the end paper: "Matt G." The book had belonged to her husband, and he must have read it while living in New York, at least half a year before he was diagnosed with cancer. She flipped back to the passage he had marked, and read it:

Somewhere and in some person, the darkness, the suffering, the chains and fetters that bind men and women must be broken down. Maybe you must be the bound one, so that your bonds may be loosed. Maybe you must be the sad one, so that in you comfort may be given. Maybe you must be the dying one, so that in you the Resurrection can be revealed. For all these things must happen in a personal way. God himself steps in among us personally; Jesus is with us quite personally…Therefore we should undertake everything we do in the spirit of service to him.

Reflecting on these words, Cynthia dismisses the idea that Matt might have had some premonition of his illness and death. But she does feel they underscore the challenge that his death leaves us. They also remind her of a prayer that gained new meaning for her during the last six months of Matt's life – the Lord's Prayer, whose final lines speak of the same readiness:

So many people pray, "Thy kingdom come; thy will be done." But how many of us actually mean it? We say it because that's what we've been taught to say, but do we *really* want God's kingdom to come? After Matt and I got married, we couldn't pray those words without crying, because we knew that it meant an end to all our selfish enjoyments, an end to the happy marriage and the children we had always wanted, an end to so many

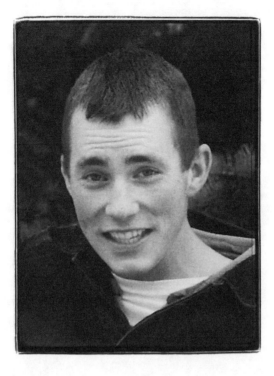

other things. We sensed what it would cost. But we really did mean it.

People tell me how deeply Matt's life affected them. They tell me that it's made them love others more, or showed them how short life is. But that makes me really angry. I think, "Wow, I lost my husband so that you can love your wife more? So that you can feel better about yourself, or about God?" Of course, I am happy for them. But to me it isn't right if the love people feel because of Matt is just wasted on themselves – if it isn't used for a greater cause. If the kingdom is going to come, it's going to cost *each* of us some kind of sacrifice. And I think a lot of people try and hide so that they're not used by God. If we ask for renewal, we have to be willing to pay the price.

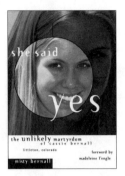

SHE SAID YES

*The Unlikely Martyrdom
of Cassie Bernall*

Misty Bernall

Foreword by Madeleine L'Engle

FEW TRAGEDIES have grabbed the public's attention in recent years as the Columbine High School massacre of April 20, 1999. And of all the stories to emerge from that day, the one that still seems to fascinate Americans most is that of Cassie Bernall, the student who was asked whether she believed in God. She answered "yes," and was then shot to death by two crazed classmates.

It was her last word, and it echoed around the globe. But it wasn't the whole story. Behind the image of the stained-glass window saint portrayed by the media was a teenager who worried about her weight, her work, and her chances of finding a boyfriend. It's a story that her mother, Misty Bernall, tells in this book with disarming honesty and compelling devotion – a story that everyone who cares about teens needs to read.

PEOPLE MAGAZINE

Far more complicated and enlightening than the tidy martyrdom imposed on Cassie after her death…
A poignant wake-up call to parents.

HARDCOVER, 160 PAGES.

**TO ORDER CALL 800-521-8011 (US),
0800 018 0799 (UK), OR 44 (0)1580 88 33 44 (EU).**

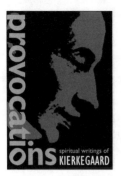

PROVOCATIONS
Spiritual Writings of Kierkegaard

Compiled and Edited
by Charles E. Moore

PRAISED AS "the most accessible Kierkegaard volume to be published in decades," *Provocations* contains a little of everything from Kierkegaard's prodigious output, including his famously cantankerous (yet humorous) attacks on what he calls the "mediocre shell" of conventional Christianity, his pithy parables, and his incisive attempts to dig through the fluff of theology and clear a way for the simple truths of the Gospel.

EUGENE PETERSON, AUTHOR
In a culture awash in religious silliness, Kierkegaard's bracing metaphors expose our mediocrities and energize us with a clarified sense of what it means to follow Jesus.

ROBERT ELLSBERG, AUTHOR
Few writers have so ably distinguished the difference between real Christianity and its many counterfeit versions.

SOFTCOVER, 464 PAGES.

**TO ORDER CALL 800-521-8011 (US),
0800 018 0799 (UK), OR 44 (0)1580 88 33 44 (EU).**

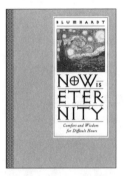

NOW IS ETERNITY

*Comfort and Wisdom
for Difficult Hours*

J. C. and C. F. Blumhardt

BAD DAYS are one thing – everyone has them now and then. But what about the darker clouds that settle over life? What about discouragement, depression, and loneliness; the trauma of separation or divorce, illness or death?

Offering something the best sympathy card cannot, this time-tested little volume reflects the stubborn faith that one day, every tear *will* be dried, and the hope that even the worst trials of human experience can be overcome with the help of God, who watches over every life.

Ideal for daily use, *Now Is Eternity* contains seventy brief meditations, with crimson titling and black text.

KARL BARTH

Blumhardt's message is a most spontaneous and penetrating word of God, and it speaks right into the need of the world.

SOFTCOVER, 70 PAGES.

TO ORDER CALL 800-521-8011 (US),
0800 018 0799 (UK), OR 44 (0)1580 88 33 44 (EU).